THE COMPLETE

GOUT

MANAGEMENT & NUTRITION GUIDE

THE COMPLETE GOUT MANAGEMENT & NUTRITION GUIDE

Empowering Strategies for Better Health

Diana Girnita, MD, PhD, FACR

with **Doug Cook,** RD, MHSc

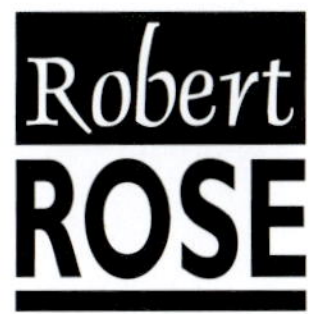

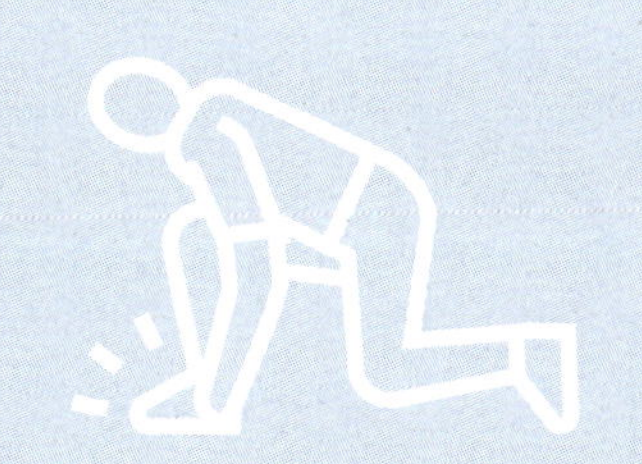

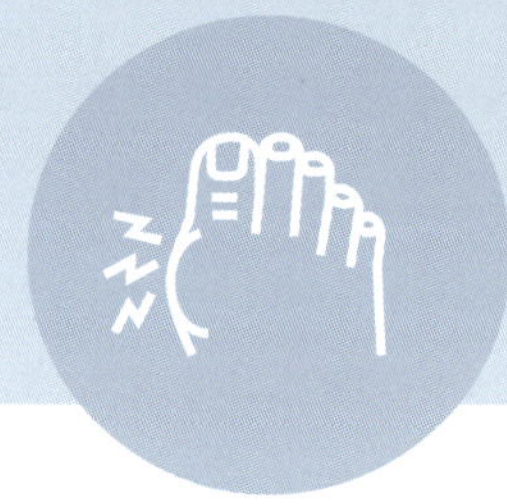

Contents

Introduction   8

PART I
EVERYTHING YOU NEED TO KNOW ABOUT GOUT   12

CHAPTER 1
Introducing Gout   13

CHAPTER 2
Diagnosing Gout   22

CHAPTER 3
Living with Gout   48

CHAPTER 4
Food Journaling and Gout-Friendly Meal Plans   92

PART II
THE RECIPES   103

CHAPTER 5
Breakfast   104

CHAPTER 6
Lunch   134

CHAPTER 7
Dinner   160

CHAPTER 8
Soups and Salads   190

CHAPTER 9
Sides   212

Recipe Sources   240

References and Resources   244

Index   250

IF YOU'VE EXPERIENCED GOUT, you'll remember it vividly. People say it is the most painful ordeal they have ever been through. Sadly, your first experience won't be a one-off incident. Without proper treatment, your attacks will continue, worsening in severity and increasing in frequency. Add to this your growing awareness that much of what you're learning about your disease seems to lack certainty. You are likely to feel as if you're swimming upstream.

Fundamentally, there are many differing opinions on when and how to treat gout, even among highly regarded experts. The complexity of the disease is significant. Physicians have been treating gout since antiquity, but for centuries they had no idea what triggered an attack. It wasn't until the 1960s that researchers identified the direct perpetrator, too much uric acid in your body.

I see the results of this uncertainty in my daily practice. Gout is a common disease, but it's likely to be misdiagnosed and/or mismanaged. A patient's first response to the symptoms is probably to book an appointment with their family physician. Unfortunately, some primary-care providers don't know how best to treat gout. They may confuse high uric acid levels in the blood with the condition. They may also be unsure about whether to treat the pain or initiate long-term therapy.

Gout is a common disease, but it's likely to be misdiagnosed and/or mismanaged.

Our current medical system also makes treatment challenging. Even if your family physician has the best intentions, they don't have time to discuss long-term management in the standard 10-minute visit. An emergency or urgent-care consultation is equally problematic, as a one-time visit doesn't include a comprehensive evaluation or follow-up.

For many reasons, which I'll explain later, making an accurate diagnosis of gout can be complicated. Basically, the earlier you begin proper treatment, the better your outcome is likely to be. If you have gout, you need to see a specialist as quickly as possible.

While experts agree on how to treat gout, they debate the impact that food and lifestyle can have in its management. One active debate revolves around the benefits of pharmaceutical interventions compared to lifestyle modifications such as changes to diet. There is no question that drugs are effective in the acute phase of an attack. They work quickly, providing immediate pain relief. But long-term management of the condition requires a more comprehensive approach.

If you are suffering from gout, it is likely you will encounter a specialist who will tell you there is no scientific evidence linking what you eat to an attack of gout—even if your experience shows a clear connection.

There are many reasons for this. One, generally, doctors have minimal education in nutrition. We have been trained to recognize and diagnose a disease, then treat it with medications. Also, there is a sad lack of "gold standard" studies linking nutrition with gout.

Usually, we as physicians do not talk to patients about nutrition or supplements, even when patients initiate the discussion. We are afraid to make recommendations, as this information is outside the rules governing the standard of care. Most of our recommendations are very general: "Don't eat too much protein. Don't drink too much alcohol. Sleep well and exercise. Avoid stress." How is that advice supposed to help patients? If we don't give patients a plan to follow, our advice is just a wish list.

Yes, medication has an important part to play in treating gout. But as a researcher and a rheumatologist who has been treating patients with gout for 10 years, I know that nutrition has a major role to play in the long-term management of gout. You can't successfully manage the disease without involving diet.

Nutrition has a major role to play in the long-term management of gout.

I became a rheumatologist via a circuitous route. In 2005, as a cardiology resident, I was invited to pursue a postdoctoral fellowship at Harvard University to study heart disease. A year later, at the University of Pittsburgh, I investigated the relationship between our genes and the immune system. One fundamental lesson I learned there is that our genes influence how our bodies react to inflammation; if you are predisposed to develop more inflammation, it is mostly because of your genes. I enjoyed my research work but, after five years, I was missing direct interaction with patients. I took the plunge and undertook further training to become a board-certified specialist in internal medicine and rheumatology.

Since then, I've evaluated many patients with gout and have learned first-hand how much misunderstanding there is about the disease as well as how frequently it is misdiagnosed and poorly managed. Over the years, patients often asked me about nutrition. I felt frustrated, as I did not have all the answers. I started to study how certain foods, supplements and lifestyle changes could affect gout. I went back to school and studied nutrition science at Stanford University, then did further research into mindfulness at the University of Massachusetts. Since then, I have spent hundreds of hours researching the topics I discuss in this book.

My practical experience made me aware of another problem. Accessing specialists in the United States is very difficult. Recognizing that patients who are in pain and need immediate help can easily wait four to six months to get an appointment with a rheumatologist, I started my own practice, Rheumatologist OnCall. Through my company, patients can reach me from their homes via telemedicine anywhere in the United States.

I wrote this book because I wanted to clarify the confusion about gout and to help people who are suffering from the disease. Gout is more than an acute attack that subsequently goes away. It's a much deeper problem involving your entire metabolism. Gout is strongly connected with numerous metabolic diseases, including obesity, diabetes, psoriasis and hypertension. Left untreated, it will leave its mark on your entire body, damaging organs such as your heart, blood vessels and kidneys.

Gout is strongly connected with numerous metabolic diseases, including obesity, diabetes, psoriasis and hypertension.

I felt compelled to write this book because I see so much unscientific information about nutrition being bandied about. These days many "experts"—some of whom have never treated a patient in their life—dispense all kinds of misguided advice across multiple social media platforms. When it comes to nutrition, I want to set the record straight. In this book, I share what I know about the scientifically proven dietary interventions that will likely help you prevent onset of gout and decrease the frequency of gout attacks.

Many patients who come to see me want to know what they can eat. That's not a simple, one-size-fits all answer, in part, because our unique genetic makeup affects how we process food. Our genes influence our immune system, raising the risk of inflammation in certain individuals. That means if someone who is genetically vulnerable eats a food that is wrong for them, it will probably spark inflammation and increase the frequency of gout attacks.

Patients know enough about nutrition to recognize that they need to change their diet and lifestyle, but they need guidance.

And that's what this book can provide. It is intended to be a bridge between nutrition and lifestyle interventions and pharmaceutical options. It recognizes that these solutions can co-exist. They should complement, not exclude each other, leading to a better outcome. With the help of this book, you can live a better life with the least amount of medication.

In this book, I tell you everything you wanted to know about gout, from how to identify the disease to the various treatments available. I also teach you about foods and their relationship with gout. You may know that certain foods can trigger a gout attack, but you may not be aware that eating other foods can help with controlling the disease. You will learn how to identify the foods and lifestyle choices that work for you—putting you in the driver's seat managing your gout.

Finally, I provide some practical tools for keeping gout at bay. These include detailed instructions on how to keep a food diary as well as a 30-day meal plan with delicious recipes.

Many factors have contributed to your gout, and no standard-issue approach is going to fix your problem. We can't cure your gout, but we can improve your quality of life and prevent the disease from further damaging your body. This book will tell you what you need to do to help you understand your condition and live a more enjoyable life.

This book is not about how to cure gout but rather how to manage it better and avoid future complications. It is intended to be a bridge between nutrition and lifestyle interventions and pharmaceutical options.

Is this book for you?

- If you are newly diagnosed with gout, this book will fully explain the condition—what it is and how you can take control over it.
- If you are a long-suffering gout patient who seems to spend too much time in severe pain, it will equip you with a fresh perspective, providing information that will help you reduce the frequency of your attacks and downscale their severity.
- If you have a family member with gout or you are caring for someone with the disease, it will help you to understand their experience and provide you with supportive tools.

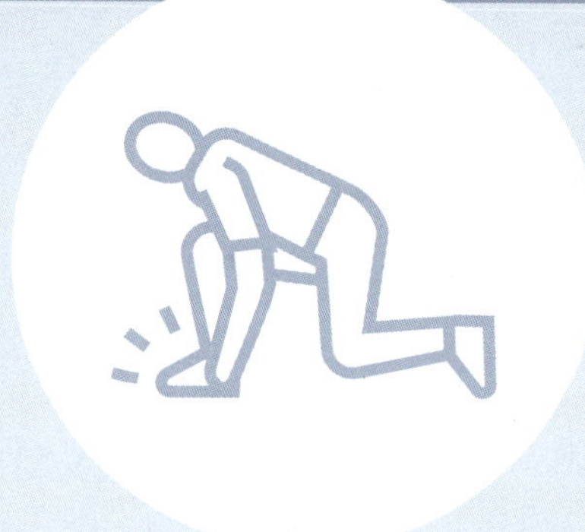

Everything You Need to Know About Gout

CHAPTER 1

Introducing Gout

What Is Gout?

Gout is a particularly painful type of arthritis that results from excessive uric acid accumulation, which causes inflammation in certain joints.

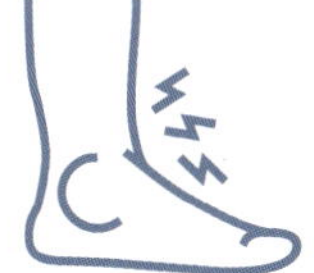

Practitioners have recognized gout for centuries but until relatively recently we didn't know what caused it. The ancient Greek physician Hippocrates called gout "the unwalkable disease." It's an apt description, as gout usually affects the big toe and foot, making mobility difficult.

It's not surprising that gout has an image problem. In the past, gout mainly affected affluent people, in particular, those whose diets were built around meat (often game) washed down with plenty of alcohol. As a result, the disease has traditionally been associated with an over-the-top lifestyle characterized by exuberant appetites. One sufferer, Benjamin Franklin, a founding father of America, fit these criteria. Attacks of gout often confined him to bed with excruciating pain. However, he maintained his sense of humor despite his misery. Playfully, he published a witty dialogue with his disease, blaming it for "outing" him as a "glutton and a tippler" and ruining his good name.

GOUT: THE DISEASE OF KINGS

There are reasons why gout has been called "disease of kings." When King Henry VIII died in 1547 at age 55, his early demise was attributed in part to gout. An excellent physical specimen in his youth, the monarch indulged his many appetites, becoming grossly obese. In his later years, he couldn't walk and needed to be carried around in a custom-built chair.

We don't know for sure if Henry VIII suffered from gout. But historians tell us that during his reign, gout was so prevalent among European nobility that it was viewed as a status symbol. However, given what we now know about the disease, it's likely that at least some of those nobles didn't have gout. They may have been suffering from other ailments. Henry VIII himself is a case in point. Many believed that he suffered from gout, while others now do not. This confirms our current understanding that gout is often misunderstood and misdiagnosed.

Many famous people throughout history have suffered from the disease. These include explorer Christopher Columbus, artist Leonardo da Vinci and composer Ludwig van Beethoven. We can't say for sure whether these individuals ate and drank to excess. What we do know, however, is that some people are more vulnerable to developing gout.

Gout Attacks

A gout attack, or flare-up, is extremely painful. It usually shows up as severe swelling that begins in a lower limb or a big toe, subsequently spreading throughout the foot. Although pain is a subjective experience and therefore challenging to define, from treating patients, I'm willing to believe a gout attack may be the most painful form of arthritis.

What triggers an attack? Fundamentally, gout results from too much uric acid in your body. When this substance accumulates, sharp crystals form in your joints. These crystals spark inflammation and pain, the symptoms of a gout attack.

Gout attacks are more likely to happen during the night, when the temperature drops. Cooler temperatures cause uric acid in the joints to form crystals. The immune system senses that change and goes on the offensive, identifying the crystals as foreign substances and dispatching cells to attack and destroy them. This creates inflammation, making your joints red, swollen and extremely painful.

GOUT ATTACKS IN THE NIGHT

Gout flare-ups usually originate at night. As room temperature drops, any uric acid crystals that have been forming crystallize in the joints, triggering inflammation. In the morning, you will be greeted by a swollen and very painful toe. It's possible your entire foot will appear red and swollen.

For more about uric acid and tophi, the crystal clusters that form when there's too much uric acid in the blood, see *Chapter 2: Diagnosing Gout*.

PODAGRA

A gout flare-up usually starts in the big toe, which appears red and swollen. This inflammation is called podagra. The pain is excruciating. The maximum intensity of a gout attack is usually reached within 24 hours. Then the pain begins to wane, usually winding down in five to seven days.

A flare-up lasts for a week or two before subsiding, sometimes on its own. Using anti-inflammatory medications (such as ibuprofen, naproxen, diclofenac, indomethacin) or steroids can help to decrease inflammation sooner.

The Many Shades of Arthritis

Gout is a form of arthritis. However, arthritis isn't an easily defined disease. The Centers for Disease Control and Prevention says the term "arthritis" describes more than 100 conditions, with a wide variety of symptoms. The most common are joint pain, swelling and stiffness. These are indicators for many disorders, which accounts for some of the confusion surrounding the condition.

In general terms, arthritis falls into the following three categories: osteoarthritis, autoimmune arthritis and *crystal-induced arthritis*. Gout is a crystal-induced arthritis in which uric acid invades specific joints and inflames them. It is helpful to understand the differences between the three kinds of arthritis.

Osteoarthritis

Osteoarthritis is the most common form of arthritis and the one people typically call "arthritis." Almost 33 million Americans suffer from the condition; women, especially those older than 50, are more likely than men to develop osteoarthritis.

Osteoarthritis (or "wear-and-tear" arthritis) is not an inflammatory arthritis.

Osteoarthritis is usually attributed to "wear and tear" on the joints. Although growing older is the greatest risk factor, arthritis is not an inevitable consequence of aging. Current research suggests that a constellation of factors, such as being overweight or experiencing repetitive trauma of the sort associated with being a professional athlete, contribute to its development, as does normal age-related deterioration. The condition is likely to worsen as you age.

Fundamentally, this arthritis results when cartilage (the tissue covering your bones where they form a joint) wears away. The first symptoms are pain and stiffness that lasts for less than 30 minutes and which especially occurs after a period of inactivity such as sleep. People rarely develop swelling or redness of their joints. To clarify, osteoarthritis is not an inflammatory arthritis.

Autoimmune Arthritis

Some other forms of arthritis are classified as autoimmune diseases. An autoimmune disease results when your immune system misfires. For various reasons (some of which we don't understand), your body's natural defense system turns against you. Instead of defending you from pathogens such as viruses or bacteria, your immune system attacks you. This creates an ongoing, exaggerated inflammatory response that eventually damages your joints and other organs, including your lungs, heart and kidneys.

Some people are genetically predisposed to develop autoimmune diseases. Having a first-degree relative in your family with an autoimmune arthritis will increase your risk of developing it in the future.

There are more than 80 autoimmune diseases, including type 1 diabetes, celiac disease and multiple sclerosis. Only some of them involve the joints. These include rheumatoid arthritis, in which your immune system primarily attacks the joints in your hands and feet; ankylosing spondylitis, which affects primarily your spine, eventually causing vertebrae to fuse; and psoriatic arthritis, in which the skin disease psoriasis eventually causes inflammation in the joints. There is also a type of autoimmune arthritis that specifically affects children, called juvenile idiopathic arthritis. As with gout, these autoimmune diseases cause inflammation in the joints and they can fluctuate from periods of activity (called flare-ups) to periods of remission.

Crystal-Induced Arthritis

In some ways, crystal-induced arthritis resembles an autoimmune condition: inflammation is precipitated by a stimulus. Basically, your immune system revs up to defend itself against something invading a joint.

However, crystal-induced arthritis is not an autoimmune arthritis. If it were, other parts of the body or organs would be affected. The most common forms of crystal-induced arthritis are gout and pseudogout. With gout, uric acid invades specific joints. Uric acid is the invader that causes inflammation in the joints. With pseudogout, calcium pyrophosphate crystals invade the joints and create inflammation. This is a major difference between crystal-induced arthritis and autoimmune arthritis. Moreover, in autoimmune arthritis, inflammation doesn't usually stop. It goes on and on, affecting not only joints but many organs, causing the entire body to suffer.

Gout Copycats

Diagnosing gout can be challenging because some other diseases have similar symptoms. Any disease that presents with red, swollen and painful joints can be mistakenly identified as gout. These include "pseudogout," psoriatic arthritis, septic arthritis, osteomyelitis and rheumatoid arthritis. For more about gout copycats, see pages 24–25 in *Chapter 2: Diagnosing Gout.*

Gout: The Most Common Form of Crystal-Induced Arthritis

Gout is the most common form of crystal-induced arthritis in the Western world. One 2017 study found that 42 million people suffer with gout worldwide. Moreover, gout incidence is increasing at a rapid rate, mostly as a result of our modern lifestyles. Between 2011 and 2018, the prevalence of gout increased from 3.6 to 5.1% in the United States. Its incidence doubled in Asian Americans, reaching 6.6% during that period. Men are more affected than women, but as women approach menopause, they also develop gout at a rate that is equal to men.

Why Gout Is on the Rise

There are many reasons why rates of gout are rising so quickly, including contemporary lifestyles and an aging population.

In general terms, lifestyle is strongly implicated in the development of all chronic disease. Overconsumption of ultraprocessed foods and sedentary behavior have been linked specifically with the so-called "obesity epidemic." Obesity is much more concerning than just being fat. It is a harbinger for the development of many other serious conditions. Being obese significantly increases the likelihood you will develop gout. (For more on modern lifestyle links with gout, see *Chapter 3: Living with Gout.*)

One of the reasons more and more people are developing gout is our longer lifespans. Merely growing older raises your risk of developing any chronic disease, several of which are directly linked with gout. Most people with gout also suffer from diseases associated with metabolic syndrome, a cluster of conditions including hypertension, obesity, abdominal fat, elevated levels of triglycerides and insulin resistance. Each of these is serious on its own; together they set the stage for more deadly diseases such as type 2 diabetes, cardiovascular disease and stroke.

The longer we live, the more time there is for uric acid to build up in the body. Also, gout is strongly linked with the health of your kidneys. As kidney function gradually decreases with age, this increases the risk of developing gout. (For more about kidneys as related to gout, see page 42.)

Who Gets Gout?

Some people are genetically predisposed to developing gout. If you have a family member suffering from the condition, you are at increased risk.

For everyone else, growing older is a risk factor on its own. The longer you live, the more likely it is that you will develop gout. Your kidneys slow down, increasing the possibility that uric acid will build up in your body. Moreover, as you age, you are increasingly likely to gain weight; obesity is a significant risk factor for the disease.

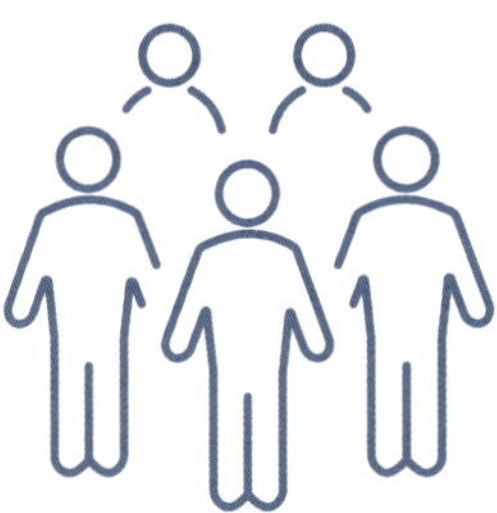

Gout Risk Factors

■ Lifestyle

As noted already, our unhealthy lifestyles also oil the wheels of gout. Many experts now link our Westernized diets, heavy in ultraprocessed foods, along with our collective tendency toward couch potato behavior, to the development of numerous chronic diseases. Gout is among them.

■ Age Is a Risk Factor

As with all chronic diseases, your risk of developing grout increases as you grow older. With aging, particularly after age 40, your kidney function declines. Sluggish kidneys contribute to uric acid buildup in your body.

■ Men Are More Prone to Gout

Men are more disposed to developing gout than women, in part because they are more likely to make poor dietary choices. This includes over-imbibing in alcohol and/or foods such as red meat and seafood known to spark uric acid production.

■ Hormones Shield Younger Women from Gout

The hormone estrogen, which tends to be abundant during women's reproductive years, provides kidney support, flushing out uric acid. Estrogen levels decline with menopause, raising the risk of developing gout.

■ A Dangerous Combination

Your genes predispose you to gout. But if you are also overweight, you are more likely to develop gout at an early age. To avoid gout, know your family history and maintain a healthy weight.

■ Diet Is Related to Gout

One 2023 study showed a clear correlation between eating ultraprocessed foods and an increased risk of developing gout. People with a genetic predisposition (a family member who has gout) were especially vulnerable to the negative effects associated with eating these foods. For more about diet considerations, see *Chapter 3: Living with Gout*.

Why Me?

Gout is linked with uric acid. Uric acid builds up in your body for two basic reasons: either your body produces too much of this waste product or for various reasons it isn't able to excrete as much as it needs to. Various factors contribute to this problem, such as your lifestyle and age, as noted above, as well as genes, gender, diet, health and kidney function.

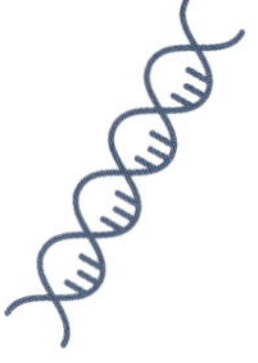

- **GENES:** Genome-wide association studies have linked more than 200 genetic variants with an increased risk of developing gout. The simplest way to assess your genetic risk is to know if you have a family member with gout.

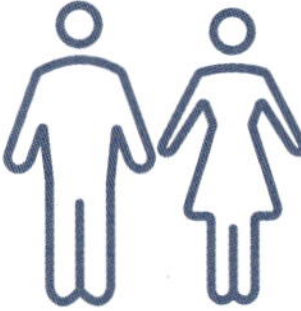

- **GENDER:** If you were born male, for much of your life you are three times more likely to suffer from gout than if you were born female. Women naturally have more estrogen, a hormone that helps their kidneys to flush out uric acid. However, as menopause approaches, their estrogen levels decline, increasing their risk of developing gout.

- **DIET:** The industrialization of our food supply plays a significant role in the rising rates of gout. Specifically, eating too much ultraprocessed food and/or animal protein has been shown to increase levels of uric acid in the body.

- **HEALTH:** Certain types of cancer, including lymphoma, leukemia and multiple myeloma, induce high cell turnover, potentially causing simultaneous cell death in multiple cells. Some chemotherapy drugs can cause normal as well as cancerous cells to rapidly die. Through complex processes, these situations can trigger a rapid increase in uric acid production, which overwhelms the kidneys, leading to gout. Having psoriasis is another risk factor for gout. This autoimmune disease can disrupt the natural process of skin cell death, increasing uric acid production.

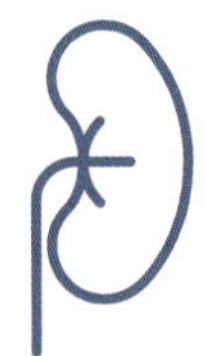

- **KIDNEY FUNCTION:** If your kidney function is poor (due to high blood pressure, diabetes or just getting older), your body may not be able to adequately eliminate uric acid.

Your specialist will look at these factors and more when considering a diagnosis of gout. For more about the reasons why some people are more likely to get gout, in particular, some common causes of hyperuricemia (high uric acid levels), see pages 32–35 in *Chapter 2: Diagnosing Gout.*

Stop Gout in Its Tracks

It's far easier and less expensive to prevent gout from occurring and to control it effectively in its early stages than it is to allow it to progress unchecked.

If someone in your family has gout, ask your primary-care provider to order an annual uric acid test for you. This test will show if your levels are remaining stable or increasing. If they are increasing, it's time to commit to the lifestyle modifications outlined in *Chapter 3: Living with Gout.*

While medications are available to manage gout, medications always come with a price, literally as well as figuratively. Drugs can be expensive. They also require regular monitoring, increasing the cost of your health care. Wouldn't you prefer to spend that money on fun activities?

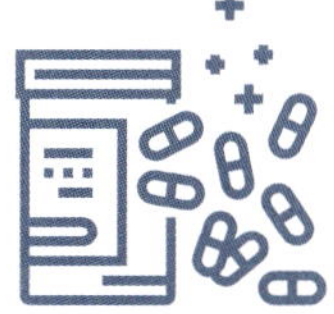

Medications also generate unpleasant side effects in many people, from minor inconveniences such as a skin rash to major health hazards, such as an increased risk of heart attack. Most people with gout have other metabolic conditions, and these are likely being treated with other pharmaceuticals, raising the risk of dangerous drug interactions. Older people are especially likely to be taking multiple prescription drugs simultaneously to treat their various conditions. Taking four or more medications regularly has been shown to increase the risk of adverse outcomes, from injuries from falls to drug reactions requiring hospital admission. "Polypharmacy" has been linked with increased mortality.

Prioritizing gout prevention or decreasing the frequency of gout attacks isn't just about avoiding pain; it's also about supporting a long and fulfilling old age.

The ongoing stress—physical as well as economic—of taking medication can also have a negative impact your overall health, potentially shortening your lifespan.

Remember, gout is not an isolated condition. Prioritizing gout prevention and decreasing the frequency of gout attacks isn't just about avoiding pain; it's also about supporting a long and fulfilling old age.

CHAPTER 2

Diagnosing Gout

IN THIS CHAPTER, we look at the ways in which gout is sometimes misdiagnosed, the signs to watch for (and the medical reasons behind those signs) and the process and tests I use to determine if my patient has gout. We also explore how gout is a metabolic disease, and further examine the causes of gout, plus we look at what tophi are and how gout and kidney disease are related. Finally, we look at some unexpected triggers for gout attacks.

As noted in *Chapter 1: Introducing Gout,* early diagnosis of gout is important. Patients first look for help when they develop gout flare-ups, as they are extremely painful. Typically, your first attack will evolve into an annual event. Gradually the frequency will increase, eventually morphing into something along the lines of monthly occurrences. On their own, these attacks will curb your ability to work and hamstring your enjoyment of life. However, repeated episodes will eventually leave their mark throughout your body.

CASE STUDY **ALEX**

One bright, sunny afternoon, Alex, a 24-year-old software engineer, walked into my office. A physically active man who loved hiking, he had been in pain for weeks. His right big toe was swollen, red and somewhat painful, and it hurt to walk, His primary-care physician suspected gout and referred him to my rheumatology office. His father had a long history of gout.

I took a history and something didn't feel right. Alex was health-conscious; he ate a balanced diet, exercised regularly and rarely drank alcohol. On further questioning, he mentioned that his skin had recently been acting out. He also noticed a few patches of dandruff in his scalp and a few red and white patches of scaly skin around his belly button and in his genital area. His nails had multiple dents and were very frail.

A few years back, he had some white, scaly patches on his elbows that resolved after applying steroid cream. I began to suspect that Alex likely had psoriasis. When I examined his right toe, I noticed that the second toe was also swollen like a sausage. At that point, I started to doubt the gout diagnosis and, instead, consider psoriatic arthritis, a form of arthritis that may occur in people with psoriasis. Its symptoms mimic those of gout.

Gout Is Easily Misdiagnosed

Unfortunately, gout is often left untreated or even misdiagnosed. Its symptoms can easily be mistaken for those of other conditions, including sprains, tendinitis or even different types of arthritis. (See *Gout Copycats,* below.)

Because it's so painful, most people experiencing a gout attack immediately seek treatment from their family physician or at an urgent-care facility. These practitioners may or may not recognize gout. However, they likely have the skills to relieve the patient's pain. Once the sufferer feels better, they are likely to forget about the attack until the next time.

The problem is, each flare-up signals that the disease is progressing. Every attack further damages the joint, which over time will be destroyed, leading to chronic pain. And there will be a next time. If left unchecked, gout will run rampant throughout your body.

Expertise Pays Off

Diagnosing and treating gout requires a specialist's expertise and the time to take a detailed inventory of the patient's history and lifestyle habits. Unfortunately, in the current health-care environment, physicians are penalized for more spending time with their patients. The health-care system values productivity—the number of patients seen in an hour—more than the quality of patient care. In addition, our current medical system is focused on treating sickness, not on preventing it from developing in the first place.

I'm a board-certified rheumatologist, with more than 20 years of training and practical experience. When patients present at my office, I carefully listen to their symptoms and look for particular signs when examining them. These will guide my next steps in getting an accurate diagnosis.

I think of myself as a kind of medical detective. My first meeting with a patient involves taking detailed notes and piecing together symptoms and signs. Then I connect the dots to make a diagnosis of gout. Once I suspect that the patient might have gout, I do a battery of tests that guide me toward the diagnosis. After confirming gout, I choose the treatments that are likely to be the most effective based on that patient's medical conditions. Each and every patient represents a unique challenge. There is no one-size-fits-all solution.

Gout Copycats

Other diseases that present with red, swollen and painful joints can be mistakenly identified as gout. These include "pseudogout," psoriatic arthritis, septic arthritis, osteomyelitis and rheumatoid arthritis.

■ Calcium Pyrophosphate Deposition (Pseudogout)

Gout can be confused with another type of arthritis, calcium pyrophosphate deposition (CPPD), formerly called pseudogout. However, the crystals that irritate the joints in CPPD are calcium phosphate crystals, not the uric acid crystals linked with gout.

Patients with this condition present with excruciating pain and swelling in their joints. However, CPPD usually affects the wrists and knees. While some patients with gout present with pain and swelling in their knees, gout predominantly affects the big toes and foot.

These diseases are difficult to differentiate based on joints affected or appearance. In each, the joints appear swollen and red, and are warm to the touch. They are also very painful. However, their triggers are different. CPPD is caused by a buildup of calcium crystals, while gout is caused by a buildup of uric acid. The only way to tell is by doing a synovial fluid analysis, which will identify whether the crystals are caused by a buildup of calcium or uric acid. A proper diagnosis is crucial, as their long-term treatments differ.

■ Psoriatic Arthritis

It's easy to confuse psoriatic arthritis with gout because it, too, attacks your toes or fingers. While painful, it is not as excruciating as gout. It targets the entire digit, making it swell up like a sausage that ballooned in the middle. The inflammation associated with psoriatic arthritis, known as dactylitis, is often described as "sausage fingers."

Interestingly, gout and psoriatic arthritis can co-exist. Some patients with psoriasis develop gout. Psoriasis causes a high rate of skin turnover, which can cause uric acid to build up.

■ Septic Arthritis

Septic arthritis is form of arthritis caused by a pathogen such as a bacteria, virus or parasite. The invader can enter a joint space via a skin breakage, through an injection or through the blood.

For example, patients with diabetes are particularly vulnerable to septic arthritis because they may suffer from peripheral neuropathy, a condition causing pain and numbness in the legs and feet. If a person

with diabetes steps on a nail or has a skin breakage in the foot area,
they may end up with an infection that affects the toes, which may
be misdiagnosed as gout. This is highly problematic. Steroids work
by suppressing the immune system, exactly what you don't want
when your body needs to fight an infection. If the toe infection is
confused with gout, the standard treatment with steroids may decrease
the power of the immune system, aggravate the infection and even
set the stage for septic shock.

Taking a careful history to differentiate gout from septic arthritis
is important. Patients with septic arthritis have high-grade fevers,
chills and night sweats. They might have a concomitant skin infection,
or have recently had pneumonia, a urinary tract infection or diarrhea.
The most reliable test to distinguish septic arthritis from gout is
analysis of the synovial fluid. If it is gout, the cultures will reveal
uric acid crystals, not a pathogen.

■ Osteomyelitis

Osteomyelitis is an infection that spreads from the skin or blood
to involve the bones near a joint. It causes a dull persistent pain and
swelling around a joint. It may be accompanied by fever and chills.
The pain can worsen with activity or pressure on the affected bone.

If osteomyelitis presents in the foot, it is likely to be mistaken for
gout. Practitioners treating patients with a history of diabetes who
experience trauma to the foot should consider osteomyelitis when
they see swelling of the toe or foot. An MRI is the best diagnostic
tool, because it will show any changes in the bone that suggest
osteomyelitis.

■ Rheumatoid Arthritis

Rheumatoid arthritis (RA) is an autoimmune condition that causes
pain and swelling in the joints. It affects joints in a symmetric and
bilateral pattern (both hands, both feet and/or both ankles at the same
time). In contrast, gout usually tackles just one joint at a time.

However, when rheumatoid arthritis affects the foot, it may be
misdiagnosed as gout. One indicator that it's not gout is when the
pain appears in both feet. If it starts in the toes, it won't be one
toe; it will be all the toes and on both feet. Another differentiator
is that RA causes a gradual onset of pain; it does not come overnight
like gout does. RA causes significant and prolonged (more than
one hour) morning stiffness, but with gout, there is no morning
stiffness and activity such as walking on the affected foot will
worsen the symptoms.

Gout Is a Metabolic Disease

I believe strongly that any patient being assessed for gout should undergo a comprehensive evaluation to help identify any associated conditions.

Gout almost never appears alone. It is considered a metabolic disease and is usually linked with conditions associated with metabolic syndrome, all of which are also on the rise.

Many doctors can provide relief from an acute gout attack, successfully taming the pain for a period of time. However, that gout flare-up is just the tip of the iceberg. Repeated episodes of inflammation can destroy the joints, leading to chronic pain and other problems. Ultimately, the disease will affect your entire body, leaving its marks not only on your joints, but also on other organs, including your blood vessels, heart and your kidneys. Over time, it will shorten your life expectancy. By 2060, it is estimated that gout mortality rates will increase by 55%.

When you have gout, treating gout attacks on their own might not be enough to change the long-term outcome or improve life expectancy. That is why it is so important to understand any other associated conditions as well.

Gout Is Part of a Package

Gout is never just one diagnosis. Most people with gout suffer with other chronic diseases, including high blood pressure, diabetes, kidney diseases, obesity, high cholesterol and/or psoriasis. Because gout is closely connected with metabolic syndrome and its constellation of conditions, patients being assessed for gout should have a comprehensive evaluation that addresses these associated diseases.

WHAT IS METABOLIC SYNDROME?

Metabolic syndrome is a cluster of medical conditions specifically related to heart disease. These medical conditions are disorders that disrupt the metabolic process. They include obesity, high blood pressure, high triglycerides, low HDL (good) cholesterol and insulin resistance.

Misdiagnosis: A Path for Complications

As discussed, gout is considered a metabolic disease. Most people with gout suffer from other chronic conditions such as high cholesterol, high blood pressure, obesity, diabetes, psoriasis or kidney disease, all of which signal that something is amiss with the metabolism.

Complications specifically associated with gout include buildup of tophi, chronic pain, heart disease and reduced life expectancy.

- **BUILDUP OF TOPHI:** Deposits of uric acid crystals known as tophi are associated with gout. They can emerge under your skin, commonly near joints such as those in the hands, feet and elbows. Tophi have the potential to erode joints, leading to bone damage and persistent pain. (See page 39 for more on tophi.)

- **CHRONIC PAIN:** Recurring attacks of gout can wear down your joints, causing significant pain and restricting movement.

- **HEART DISEASE:** Elevated uric acid levels affect more than your joints; they can also promote inflammation in your blood vessels, increasing the risk of heart ailments and even strokes.

- **REDUCED LIFE EXPECTANCY:** High uric acid levels are commonly associated with heart and kidney diseases. These conditions can negatively affect your quality of life and how long you will live. Recent research links keeping uric acid levels within a healthy range with longevity.

If left untreated, gout will ravage your body, often in unexpected ways. An initially nagging pain in your foot can cascade into a slew of more dire health concerns affecting not just joints but other organs, including the heart and kidneys.

The Rabbit Hole of Self Diagnosis

If you wake up with a painful and swollen toe, "Dr. Google" may be the first place you look to discover what might be wrong. There are many reasons for this. Getting an appointment with your doctor can take time, or you may be worried about the cost. And, of course, on-line searching is so easy to do. Just typing in "toe pain" will produce several options, along with potential solutions. You may be tempted to try some of these remedies before calling a medical professional. If you have gout, that would be a mistake.

As noted, many conditions look similar to gout. The problem is, their treatments differ and mistreatment can have negative effects. For instance, if your toe pain is the result of an infection rather than gout, antibiotics are required. Treating it with a steroid, a gout-friendly medication, is exactly the wrong thing to do. These medications suppress the immune system, potentially worsening the infection. They might even set the stage for sepsis, a generalized infection that can be life-threatening.

If gout is the source of your pain, you need to tamp down the inflammation with a nonsteroidal anti-inflammatory drug (NSAID) or a steroid medication and then investigate long-term treatment to keep the condition under control. Although the instinct may be simply to respond to the pain, it is important to remember that untreated gout will take a heavy toll on your body.

When confronted with a complex and potentially deceptive ailment such as gout, consulting with a rheumatologist or other specialist can make all the difference.

CASE STUDY — GEORGE

George's story highlights the value of timely diagnosis.

One morning, George woke up to a red and swollen ankle that was throbbing with pain. An avid cyclist, he immediately assumed he'd injured himself while riding his bike. His first solution was to try some home remedies. These included splinting, icing and applying heat to his ankle. When that didn't help, he went to urgent care. There, he was advised to continue icing, take ibuprofen for three to four days and follow up with his family physician.

The pain and swelling persisted. Three days after his urgent-care visit, he saw his primary-care physician. The physician ordered x-rays to rule out a fracture and advised George to continue with ibuprofen for the next five days. George's pain improved somewhat but the ankle remained swollen. At that point, his primary-care physician referred him to me.

After reviewing his medical history, I advised George that we should take some synovial fluid to rule out infection. When that fluid revealed uric acid crystals, the diagnosis was clear: George had gout. We initiated treatment. This was George's first attack of gout and he became my patient. When he was correctly diagnosed and began his gout-targeted treatment, his condition quickly improved.

Pinpointing Gout: Taking a History and Using Power Tools

Diagnosing and treating gout requires a specialist's expertise and the time to take a detailed inventory of the patient's history and lifestyle habits. Every patient represents a unique challenge. No one solution will work for everyone. Many different factors set the stage for gout, from genes and being overweight to prescription medications and poor lifestyle choices.

Simple questions can help to streamline a diagnosis. These include:

- Does any member of your family suffer from gout?

- What foods do you usually eat?

- How much alcohol do you drink?

- Do you suffer from other chronic conditions, such as heart disease, diabetes, obesity, kidney disease, lymphoma, cancer or multiple myeloma?

- Are you taking any of the following medications: diuretics, blood pressure medications, chemotherapy drugs?

Once I've taken a detailed patient history, I use my power tools—from basic laboratory tests to the most advanced imaging tests—to zero in on whether gout is the source of the patient's problems.

Reliable First Steps

- When gout is suspected, I usually test the patient's *uric acid level* first. If this blood test shows that the uric acid level is higher than 6.5 mg/dL, it is considered abnormal, increasing the odds that you might have gout. As noted, however, gout is complex. Not everyone with high blood levels of uric acid develops gout.

- If I suspect a gout attack, one thing I'm always looking for is *elevated markers of inflammation*. Markers of inflammation will be high during a flare-up. They can be measured by testing sedimentation rate and C-reactive protein (CRP). During a flare-up, sedimentation rate will rapidly increase and remain high for a relatively long period of time. CRP is a protein produced by the liver in response to inflammation. It quickly increases with inflammation and decreases equally quickly when the inflammation abates.

MORE TESTS
See also page 36, *More Testing for Proving Gout,* and the table on page 38 for *Lab and Imaging Tests Used to Diagnose Gout.*

- I want to know *how well the patient's kidneys are functioning.* (This can be measured by creatinine level and estimated glomerular filtration rate.) Poor kidney function may cause high uric acid levels. If uric acid is not properly eliminated from your body, it raises the risk of developing gout.

- I also order tests to evaluate for *liver enzymes* and *insulin resistance* (hemoglobin A1c) to assess whether diabetes is a concern.

- Based on the patient's family and personal history, I might also order *genetic tests.* For instance, Asian patients can have certain HLA genes that can result in severe side effects if allopurinol therapy is used. If you are Asian, I highly recommend being tested for the HLA-B 5801 allele before taking allopurinol.

A CAVEAT

Although a uric acid test is the most common diagnostic for gout, it is not infallible. If the test is obtained during an attack, the numbers might be low, as inflammation proteins and free steroids in the blood will increase the excretion of uric acid. On the other hand, high levels of uric acid do not necessarily mean gout.

CASE STUDY — JEREMY

Based on blood tests that showed slightly high levels of uric acid, Jeremy had been diagnosed with gout five years before he saw me. He was faithfully taking the drug allopurinol, a classic and effective treatment for gout, but his condition had not improved. Eventually, he decided to seek a second opinion.

When I saw him, Jeremy's attacks were still persistent. Despite additional treatment with anti-inflammatories and steroids from time to time, he was still having gout attacks every three to four months. His left toe was definitely swollen. It looked like a sausage.

I was unable to get synovial fluid from the toe, so I ordered x-rays and a special type of CT scan (called a dual energy CT), neither of which revealed any uric acid crystals in the joint. Jeremy did, however, have high levels of inflammation. He told me that he frequently had eczema in his scalp and behind his ears. When I looked, I determined that his rash was actually psoriasis. That led me to a more likely diagnosis of psoriatic arthritis rather than gout (see page 24).

What Is Uric Acid and How Is It Produced?

Imagine enjoying your favorite meal: shrimp cocktail, steak and a delicious cake with a scoop of vanilla ice cream for dessert, washed down with a glass of ice-cold beer. As you consume each tasty bite, your body begins the complex process of converting that meal into energy.

Some of those tasty treats contain chemical compounds called *purines*. When our bodies metabolize purines, waste products including excess water and carbon dioxide are produced. One of these waste products is uric acid.

However, food is not the only source of purines. Purines are also produced when our cells break down, a natural process at all stages of life. A special enzyme, xanthine oxidase, transforms these purines into uric acid. About one-third of our daily uric acid production will be eliminated through the intestines (in stool), while two/thirds is eliminated through the kidneys.

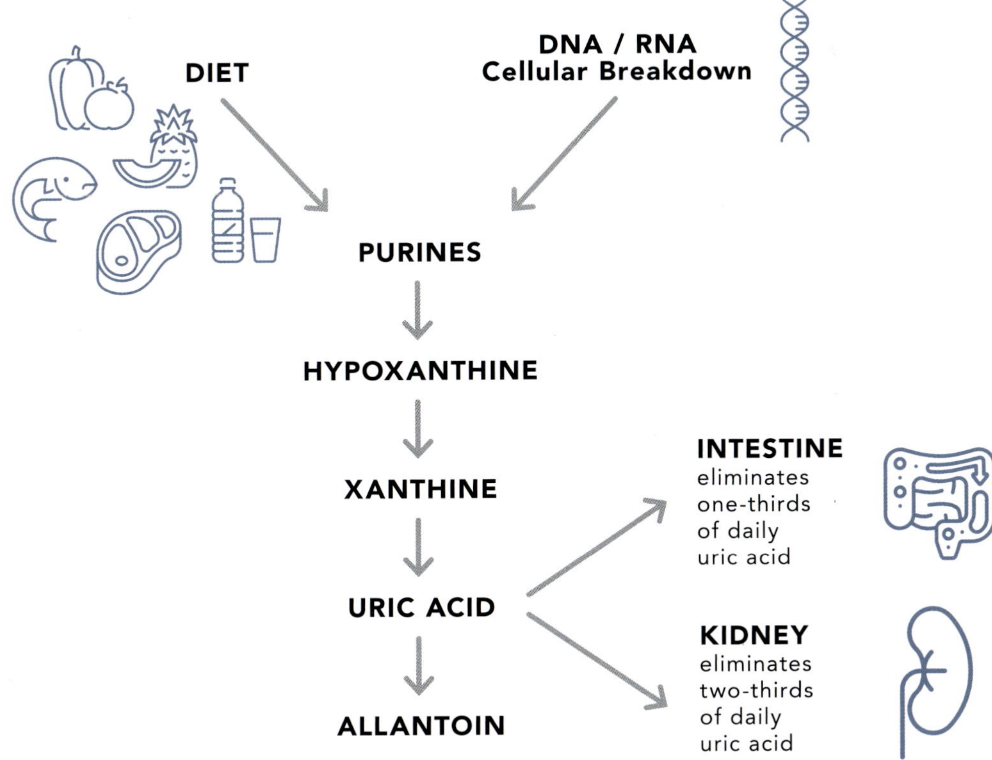

Uric acid production and metabolism in the body. Purines can result from two sources: food and cellular breakdown (cells dying). Under the action of an enzyme (xanthine oxidase), purines are transformed through a few steps into uric acid that will be eliminated though the intestine or kidneys. In humans, uric acid is the end metabolite of the purine metabolism. However, in some animal species (except mammals, including humans), plants and bacteria, there is an additional step of the uric acid metabolism, when under a certain enzyme called uricase, the uric acid is converted to allantoin. In human, this step can only happen under the action of certain medications.

Hyperuricemia

HIGH URIC ACID LEVELS

Consistently high uric acid levels are directly connected to kidney disease. They are also linked with diabetes, obesity and high cholesterol, among the cluster of conditions included in the condition known as metabolic syndrome.

Hyperuricemia is the medical term for consistently high blood levels of uric acid. Everyone is vulnerable to having high uric acid levels on occasion—for instance, when taking certain medications—even if they don't have gout. However, if your levels consistently exceed 6.5 mg/dL, you have hyperuricemia.

Hyperuricemia is a precondition for gout. However, having hyperuricemia doesn't mean you have gout. Even so, everyone with gout has high blood levels of uric acid at some point.

Persistent hyperuricemia has two main causes: either your body is producing too much uric acid, or your kidneys are not excreting enough of the uric acid you produce.

Common Causes of Hyperuricemia

High levels of uric acid in your blood are commonly caused by overproduction of uric acid and/or decreased uric acid elimination.

Overproduction of Uric Acid

Some people produce more uric acid than others. The reasons for this include genes, certain diseases and some medical treatments.

- GENES: Having certain genetic variants increases the likelihood that you will produce too much uric acid. We can easily evaluate this risk by determining if a parent or close relative has gout.

Hyperuricemia is a precondition for gout. However, having hyperuricemia doesn't mean you have gout.

If you have a genetic predisposition to gout, eating many high-purine foods that increase uric acid production will increase the risk of developing gout at a younger age.

- **CERTAIN DISEASES:** Psoriasis is associated with excess uric acid production. This is due to the rapid skin cell turnover associated with the condition, which generates purines, raising uric acid levels.

  Some types of cancer can also lead to increased uric acid levels. When cancer cells break down rapidly, they release purines, which the body converts to uric acid. This phenomenon is most intense in cancers with high cell turnover, including leukemia, lymphoma and multiple myeloma.

- **SOME MEDICAL TREATMENTS:** Cancer treatments such as chemotherapy can speed up cell death, resulting in a sudden surge in uric acid production.

Decreased Uric Acid Elimination

For various reasons, some people cannot excrete uric acid as efficiently as they should. These include poor kidney function, some diseases, dehydration and certain medications.

- **POOR KIDNEY FUNCTION:** More than 70% of the uric acid your body produces is excreted by your kidneys. If your body can't effectively eliminate the uric acid you produce, you will develop hyperuricemia. This can happen when your kidneys aren't functioning as well as they should be. For numerous reasons, people with kidney failure have a decreased capacity to eliminate waste products, including uric acid.

- **SOME DISEASES:** Certain conditions, including hypertension, psoriasis, obesity and cardiovascular disease, are associated with increased uric acid levels, most likely due to poor elimination. Increased uric acid in the blood seems to be correlated with an increased risk of developing hypertension and heart diseases.

- **DEHYDRATION:** If you're dehydrated, you won't excrete uric acid as quickly as you should. When your body is dehydrated, you don't produce as much urine. That means there is less fluid to dilute and excrete uric acid, increasing its concentration in the urine. Over time, this can lead to higher blood levels of uric acid, increasing the risk of kidney stones, as well as gout.

- **CERTAIN MEDICATIONS:** See the following pages for medications that may increase uric acid or interfere with its excretion.

Some Medications Can Increase Uric Acid

When a patient presents with the possibility of having gout, it's important to know the medications they are taking. Drugs can affect uric acid levels by raising uric acid blood levels and/or interfering with the body's ability to excrete it. Although medications are useful in controlling other health conditions, they can trigger attacks of gout.

At times, certain medications can elevate uric acid levels. These include aspirin, diuretics, ACE inhibitors, chemotherapy and immunosuppressive medications.

- **ASPIRIN:** Aspirin is one of the world's oldest and most frequently used medications. It readily available without a prescription, but cardiologists often prescribe low-dosage versions (75 to 150 mg daily) to protect against heart attacks. These low doses can potentially trigger gout flare-ups.

  Interestingly, research has shown that larger doses of aspirin (exceeding 2,000 mg daily) might reduce uric acid levels. However, this potential benefit comes with a caveat. Increased dosage raises the risk of adverse effects such as gastric ulcers or hemorrhages. Therefore, increasing aspirin intake solely to manage gout is *not recommended.*

- **DIURETICS:** These medications, commonly referred to as "water pills," aid in flushing out surplus fluids from the body. They are frequently prescribed for conditions such as high blood pressure and heart failure. Certain diuretics, notably hydrochlorothiazide and furosemide, can elevate uric acid levels, heightening the possibility of a gout flare-up.

  Not all diuretics raise the risk of triggering gout. Those known as potassium-sparing diuretics, such as spironolactone, are not as likely to raise uric acid levels.

- **ACE INHIBITORS:** ACE (angiotensin converting enzyme) inhibitors are a class of drugs frequently used to treat high blood pressure and heart failure. Most are considered safe for those with gout. However, some ACE inhibitors, such as captopril and lisinopril, may cause a minor increase in uric acid levels. These variations are often negligible and don't typically trigger gout symptoms in most individuals. Generally, their benefits exceed any potential risks.

- **CHEMOTHERAPY:** Some chemotherapy drugs can induce rapid cell destruction. This can abruptly elevate uric acid levels in the bloodstream, potentially triggering gout.

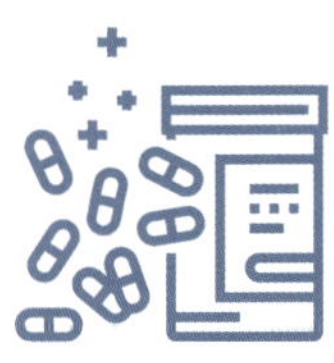

<table>
<tr><td colspan="2" align="center">UNDERSTANDING YOUR MEDICATION</td></tr>
<tr><td align="center">Medications that
Cause Gout</td><td align="center">Medications that
Do Not Cause Gout</td></tr>
<tr><td align="center">Low-dose aspirin</td><td align="center">High-dose aspirin</td></tr>
<tr><td align="center">Thiazide diuretics</td><td align="center">Potassium-sparing diuretics</td></tr>
<tr><td align="center">Loop diuretics</td><td align="center">ACE inhibitors</td></tr>
<tr><td align="center">Chemotherapy</td><td></td></tr>
<tr><td align="center">Immunosuppressants</td><td></td></tr>
</table>

CASE STUDY — RAFAEL

Rafael, a 65-year-old retired civil engineer, has always been dedicated to maintaining a balanced lifestyle. He embraces a wholesome diet, avoids alcohol and prioritizes regular physical activity. However, during a routine checkup six months before seeing me, he was diagnosed with hypertension. Consequently, his primary-care physician initiated a treatment regimen combining hydrochlorothiazide and lisinopril.

Unexpectedly, over a short span of six weeks, Rafael grappled with three agonizing gout episodes. These flare-ups were a conundrum for him; although he was aware of his father's history with gout, Rafael had never personally experienced any related symptoms. These unexpected episodes encroached upon his daily activities, hindering his morning walks and spending quality time with his grandchildren.

Upon evaluation, Rafael's doctor discovered an alarmingly elevated uric acid level in Rafael's blood, measuring 11 mg/dL. This finding hinted at gout, prompting a referral to my rheumatology clinic.

After an extensive review of his health records and current medications, I identified hydrochlorothiazide as the likely agent elevating his uric acid levels and triggering gout. I immediately liaised with his primary-care physician to address this probable medication-related setback.

Rafael's doctor transitioned him from the previous medication combination to amlodipine. With this adjustment, Rafael's gout episodes subsided, enabling him to seamlessly resume his vibrant lifestyle free from discomfort.

- **IMMUNOSUPPRESSIVE MEDICATIONS:** These drugs are often administered to organ transplant recipients or those managing autoimmune conditions. They include cyclosporine and tacrolimus, predominantly used to regulate the immune system with the goal of preventing rejection in organ transplants. They can increase uric acid levels.

In summary, while medications can be indispensable for treating various conditions, they may also trigger gout. If you are taking medication and experience symptoms of gout, consult your doctor. You may need to review and possibly adjust your medication regimen.

More Testing for Proving Gout

It takes more than a high blood level of uric acid to diagnose gout. In some cases of gout, uric acid can be normal or even low.

If one of your joints is swollen during a gout attack, your doctor may choose to take some fluid from the affected joint. A synovial fluid analysis test is important because it identifies crystals associated with gout.

In various other situations, imaging tests may also be used to confirm a gout diagnosis. These include x-rays, ultrasound and dual energy computerized tomography (CT) scans.

Synovial Fluid Analysis

When a joint is swollen, red and hot, and gout is suspected, the best way to get an accurate diagnosis is to take a small sample of the synovial fluid. Synovial fluid, also known as joint fluid, is a liquid that is essential for the health and proper function of your joints. It acts as a lubricant, much like the oil that lubricates the engine of your car, making it easier for your joints to move smoothly.

This procedure is known as arthrocentesis. We introduce a needle into the joint, aspirating some of the synovial fluid. Then we examine the sample under a special microscope. The presence of needle-shaped crystals confirms the presence of uric acid in the joints, establishing a definitive diagnosis of gout.

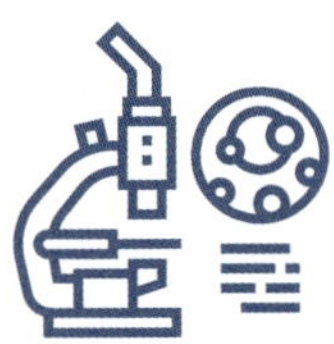

Imaging Tests

For various reasons, some patients hesitate to have needles. In these cases, imaging tests are called for. We have numerous imaging tools at our disposal, including old standbys such as x-rays. Newer imaging tools such as ultrasound and dual energy CT are noninvasive and more precise than x-rays for establishing a diagnosis of gout.

X-rays

X-rays are often used to diagnose gout, although in gout's early stages, their primary function is to rule out other possibilities. However, if someone has been suffering from undiagnosed gout for a long time, x-rays can be useful, as some characteristic findings may be observed. These include soft tissue swelling, tophi and bone erosion.

- **SOFT TISSUE SWELLING:** An acute gout attack might appear on an x-ray as swelling around the joint. It should be noted, however, that joint swelling is associated with many other conditions.

- **TOPHI:** As gout progresses, uric acid crystals may accumulate in joints and soft tissues, forming tophi (see more at page 39 and below). Tophi around the joints can damage bones, leading to "punched-out" erosions (holes in the bones) that show up on x-rays.

- **BONE EROSION:** If someone has been suffering from gout for a decade or so, x-rays will reveal a loss of bone, which means the condition is advanced.

Ultrasound

Ultrasound is often used to diagnose and monitor gout. It is a useful tool because it has the capacity to identify specific features of gout, including a double contour sign, tophi, erosions and synovitis and effusion.

- **DOUBLE CONTOUR SIGN:** This indicator, which is a powerful signal of gout, appears as an abnormal bright band on the surface of the cartilage. It reveals uric acid deposits on the cartilage.

- **TOPHI:** Tophi can show up on ultrasound as nodules with a hazy appearance within the joint space or in the soft tissues around it.

- **EROSIONS:** Bone erosions are seen in patients with long-term, chronic gout.

- **SYNOVITIS AND EFFUSION:** Gout can cause joint inflammation (synovitis) and excess fluid in the joint (effusion); these show up on ultrasound.

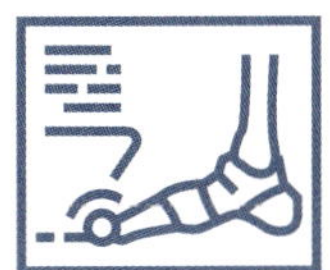

Dual Energy CT

One of the most exciting developments in gout diagnosis is dual energy CT. It is a game changer. This advanced imaging technique uses two different x-ray beams to capture super-detailed images of your body. This is especially helpful because it can visualize the exact location of the uric acid deposits in the joints, which might not show up in standard imaging procedures.

Here's how it works. When the computerized tomography (CT) scan is performed, the two x-ray beams pass through the body. Different tissues, including uric acid crystals, absorb these x-rays differently.

Dual energy CT is a powerful tool for diagnosing gout because it is accurate, noninvasive, efficient and prognostic.

- ACCURATE: This test provides a precise picture of uric acid deposits, even when they're not visible with regular imaging techniques.

- NONINVASIVE: Dual energy CT doesn't require incisions or injections; that makes it a more comfortable and patient-friendly process.

- EFFICIENT: It's fast and efficient, aiding in quicker diagnosis and treatment planning.

- PROGNOSTIC: By revealing the extent of uric acid crystal buildup, dual energy CT can help to evaluate current management strategies, guiding future treatment decisions.

LAB AND IMAGING TESTS USED TO DIAGNOSE GOUT	
Blood test	Complete cell count Renal panel Liver panel Uric acid Sedimentation rate C-Reactive protein Hemoglobin A1c
Synovial fluid	Cell Count Culture Crystals
Imaging	X-rays Ultrasound Dual energy CT

What Are Tophi?

Have you have ever noticed a small, oddly shaped bump under someone's skin, maybe on their fingers, toes or even the back of an elbow? If so, you might have observed what's known as a "tophus" (plural "tophi"). They might sound as if they're from another planet, but tophi are an important component of gout. These crystal clusters form when there's too much uric acid in the body.

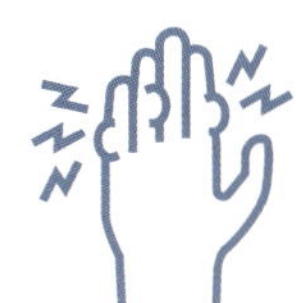

In simple terms, tophi are tiny deposits of uric acid crystals that form under the skin. Picture millions of tiny, sharp, sugarlike crystals bunched up together. They are usually white or yellow in color and, interestingly, are not tender or painful in their early stages.

Common Locations for Tophi

Although tophi can appear in various parts of your body, they are usually found around the joints—the parts of your body where two bones come together. Places where you might expect to find tophi include your fingers and toes, elbows, ankles and ears (usually on the outer edge of the ear).

Initially tophi might not be too troublesome, but over time they can become a problem. As they grow larger or increase in number, tophi exert pressure on the surrounding tissue, causing discomfort.

If tophi are not treated, they can cause long-term damage.

Imagine walking around all day with a small stone in your shoe. Initially, it might not bother you much, but if your foot continues to rub on the stone, it will start to hurt. During a gout flare, the area around a tophus can become inflamed and similarly painful.

TOPHI ARE A HARBINGER OF GOUT

Surprisingly, tophi can develop independently of a gout flare, sometimes appearing years before gout ever shows its face. This phenomenon is more prevalent in women, individuals with chronic kidney disease, and those using diuretic medications. However, the presence of tophi always announces the onset of gout.

If you notice any bumps on your ears or elbows, or around your joints, report them to your physician, who can help you to better understand these changes.

TOPHI AND KIDNEY DISEASE

The more tophi you have throughout your body, the more likely you are to develop kidney disease (see page 42).

If tophi are not treated, they can cause long-term damage. Their growth leads to swelling of the tissue surrounding the joints, bone destruction, deformity and eventually loss of movement, all of which can lead to chronic pain. When tophi grow in multiple spots on the body, chronic tophaceous gout can result (see below).

Left to grow without restriction, very large tophi will stretch the skin to the point where they cause damage. Eventually, the skin will break open, releasing a chalky white material, setting the stage for infection to develop.

EARLY TREATMENT IS CRUCIAL

Don't leave gout untreated. After many years it will most likely evolve to its chronic form, which is very hard to treat.

Chronic Tophaceous Gout

Chronic tophaceous gout is the advanced stage of tophi growth. It is the most severe form of gout. Left unchecked, tophi aren't just innocent uric acid crystal deposits. They're troublemakers who stir up a chronic inflammatory response in your body.

Imagine tophi as an invading army setting up camp in a peaceful town, causing chaos and disrupting the daily harmony. These infiltrators make their way into your body tissues and your joints, triggering inflammation. This persistent inflammation, combined with the physical presence of tophi, results in enlargement and deformation of the affected areas. Within your joints, tophi wreak havoc on your bones and cartilage, leading to pain, the loss of joint function and restricted mobility.

Imagine tophi as an invading army setting up camp in a peaceful town, causing chaos and disrupting the daily harmony.

But here's the curveball: this ongoing damage to tissues can often play tricks on us, mimicking other medical conditions. For example, when your finger or toe swells due to tophi, it might be mistaken for a condition called dactylitis, often associated with psoriatic arthritis or other forms of autoimmune arthritis (see page 24). This situation can easily lead to misdiagnosis and needless treatments.

My patient Jeremy (see page 30) is a case in point. Before seeing me, he had been treated with allopurinol for what was believed to be gout. When his toe swelling did not improve, I was quickly able to determine that his swollen joint was dactylitis resulting from psoriatic arthritis. However, because of the misdiagnosis, his treatment was delayed, leading to damaged foot tendons.

Even more worrisome, the destructive changes linked to tophaceous gout can be mistaken for a serious bone infection known as osteomyelitis (see page 25). In severe cases, this confusion can lead to unnecessary amputation of affected digits.

The good news is, if you vigilantly monitor for tophi and keep uric acid levels in check, you can catch chronic tophaceous gout early and thwart its progression. Collaborating with a health-care provider who understands gout can be your ticket to preventing the complications associated with disease development, safeguarding your quality of life.

Polyarticular Gout

Gout can easily evolve from a condition affecting a single joint to one that causes pain in joints throughout your body. This is *polyarticular gout,* and it is a situation you want to do your best to avoid.

Some patients experience gout in multiple joints simultaneously.

Another scenario involves the pain and inflammation jumping from joint to joint in a matter of days, weeks or even months. The experience is like riding a roller coaster. Once the pain is resolved in one joint, it jumps to another. It's important to take this joint hopping seriously.

Over time, the attacks will become more frequent, more painful and longer lasting.

GOUT IS A PARTY ANIMAL

Your big toe (or maybe your knee) is "party central" for about 80% of gout's first-time guests. These guests usually don't stick around for long and don't return for a few months. Just when you think they have left forever, they surprise you with a return visit, often adding another joint like your ankle to their outing.

Gout and Your Kidneys

If your kidneys are not functioning properly, your body's ability to excrete uric acid will suffer. This will increase uric acid in the blood, raising the risk of developing gout. When you have gout, your kidney function begins to decline. This deterioration can be acute or chronic.

Your kidneys need to be healthy to stay on top of gout. Your kidneys are a highly efficient waste-management system. They filter your blood, separating the good stuff your body needs to maintain, such as nutrients and water, from the waste that needs to be eliminated. This waste includes uric acid, most of which is filtered and cleared out in your urine.

Good dietary habits such as staying well hydrated, eating a nutritious diet and keeping salt and sugar to a minimum support kidney health. Steering clear of toxins, as in avoiding smoking, is also advised.

If you are overweight or obese, or have high blood pressure or diabetes, you need to pay extra attention to your kidneys. Having regular checkups that include lab tests is important. These can identify if your condition is compromising how well your kidneys function. Medications also affect your kidneys. Starting any new medication requires blood tests to check kidney function.

Your kidneys naturally slow down as you age. When your kidneys aren't functioning as well as they should be, your body may not be effectively eliminating uric acid, raising your risk of developing gout.

CASE STUDY — JAKE

Jake was a 45-year-old man living in Arizona. He worked as a landscaper, spending a great deal of time in the hot and arid outdoors. While working, he often sweated profusely but, unfortunately, he wasn't careful about keeping himself well hydrated. He constantly needed to pee, often experiencing a twinge of pain and seeing something that looked like sand grains and a little blood in his urine. One day, Jake felt a sudden, severe pain in his right side of his body. He went to the emergency room, where they took blood and ordered a non-contrast-enhanced CT scan.

The ER doctor came back with the results. His uric acid level was greater than 10 mg/dL. While his urine showed no signs of infection, it did show some crystals. Even worse, his CT scan showed a 10 mm kidney stone. Jake recalled that one year previously, he had experienced pain and swelling in his left big toe. The pain was so severe that he could barely walk for a week.

The ER doctor told Jake that he most likely had gout. Excess uric acid caused not only his previous attack in his foot, but also the kidney stone. The discovery of kidney stones was a warning sign. It prompted Jake to act before his condition got out of control. It was time for Jake to start treatment for gout. This included drinking more water, consuming a low-purine diet and taking medication to lower his uric acid levels and alkalinize his urine.

Uric Acid Kidney Stones

Another manifestation of excess uric acid is the development of uric acid kidney stones. When uric acid crystals concentrate and accumulate in the urine, they form this particular kind of kidney stone. In some cases, kidney stone formation can predate joint pain from gout, acting as a warning sign of the impending condition.

What Causes Uric Acid Stones?

Two key factors contribute to the formation of uric acid stones: high uric acid concentration in urine, and persistently acidic urine (low pH).

A persistently low urine pH (less than 5.5) creates an environment where uric acid is more likely to precipitate and form crystals that will come together and form stones.

Predisposing Medical Conditions

Certain medical conditions can cause chronically elevated uric acid production, predisposing individuals to form uric acid stones. These include:

- Gout
- Polycythemia vera
- Chronic diarrhea
- Type 2 diabetes mellitus
- Metabolic syndrome

Symptoms of Uric Acid Stones

Clinical presentation of uric acid stones often includes:

- Acute onset of back pain (often in your flank, the area between your upper abdomen and lower back)
- Increased pain and frequency during urination
- Occasional presence of blood in urine
- Reduced urine flow
- Observable "sand" or "gravel" in the urine

HOT DRY CLIMATES CAN TRIGGER URIC ACID STONES

Uric acid stones make up only 5 to 10% of urinary tract stones. However, in hot, arid climates, where low urine volume and acidic urine pH are more common due to dehydration, this proportion can soar to over 40%.

Mr. Johnson, a 62-year-old retired accountant, presented with severe pain on the right side of his back, which he'd been experiencing for a few days. He described the pain as sharp, constant and radiating toward his lower back, and reported that it had been gradually getting worse.

Two years before, Mr. Johnson had been diagnosed with polycythemia vera, a condition characterized by the excessive production of red blood cells. His current symptoms were worrisome enough that he was admitted to hospital, where several diagnostic tests were performed. A blood test revealed an elevated uric acid level (above 15 mg/dL). His kidney function showed significant deterioration since the previous month.

A urinalysis showed numerous uric acid crystals. Connecting the dots, it became clear that Mr. Johnson's current problems were related to his polycythemia vera, which causes rapid cell destruction that triggers uric acid production.

Mr. Johnson was diagnosed with acute uric acid nephropathy, most likely because the capacity of his kidneys to eliminate the excessive uric acid caused by polycythermia vera was overwhelmed. Prompt treatment focused on hydration and medications to stop the overproduction of uric acid. In a few months, his kidney function returned to normal.

Detecting Uric Acid Stones

Uric acid stones do not show up on regular x-rays. They are radiolucent, meaning they are transparent to radiation. A non-contrast-enhanced CT scan is the preferred imaging test to establish their presence.

What does the presence of uric acid stones mean for treatment? For patients with an established diagnosis of gout, the presence of uric acid stones suggests the following course of action:

- Uric acid levels must be managed more aggressively. The formation of stones indicates an ongoing issue with the body's ability to properly metabolize uric acid.

- Increased vigilance and adjustments to treatment are necessary to prevent further stone formation.

Acute Uric Acid Nephropathy

In certain situations, as with cancers, lymphomas, leukemia or
polycythemia vera, where many cells are destroyed simultaneously,
many purines are produced. Consequently, the uric acid production
becomes too much for the kidneys to eliminate. In these situations,
the overproduction of uric acid can cause an "acute" or immediate
deterioration in kidney function.

Patients may present to the hospital with pain in the side of their
back. The tests will detect a lot of uric acid crystals in their urine.
The rapid surge in excess uric acid (blood concentration above
15 mg/dL) is known as acute uric acid nephropathy.

Chronic Urate Nephropathy

Chronic urate nephropathy is a type of kidney disease that can
develop in patients with long-standing gout. Over time, uric
acid crystals slowly deposit in the kidneys, causing chronic
inflammation in the tissue. This process resembles the formation
of tophi in other parts of the body. This can lead to scarring of
the kidney tissue and chronic kidney disease, with a slow decline
in kidney function.

This form of kidney disease is particularly challenging to
diagnose. The urine may appear normal, sometimes with traces
of protein in the urine. Patients do not report much pain. However,
the more tophi in other parts of your body, the higher your chances
of developing kidney disease.

Unexpected Triggers for Gout Attacks

Traditional wisdom links gout attacks with overindulgence in
alcohol and food. Yes, certain foods and beverages can trigger
flare-ups; see *Chapter 3: Living with Gout*. However, there are
numerous other factors that can raise your risk of having a gout
attack. These include physical trauma, dehydration, previous
degenerative change, obesity, vaccination, hospitalization and/or
surgery, lower temperatures and extreme dieting.

- **PHYSICAL TRAUMA:** When you are injured or suffer repetitive
  minor trauma, your body signals a need for repair. Your immune
  system rides to the rescue by producing inflammation, which
  calms down once the injury has healed. However, if uric acid
  crystals are residing in your joints, your immune system goes
  into high gear, overdosing with inflammation, which can trigger
  a gout attack. Uric acid crystals are most likely to collect in areas
  where there has been a prior injury, which can be as minor as the
  irritation developing from wearing shoes that are too tight.

- **PREVIOUS DEGENERATIVE CHANGE:** Joints experiencing degenerative changes such as those from osteoarthritis are prone to uric acid crystals, increasing the likelihood of a flare.

- **DEHYDRATION:** Being dehydrated raises the risk of a gout flare-up. When our bodies are dehydrated, there may not be enough water to properly dilute uric acid through urine. In that situation, excess uric acid can accumulate, setting the stage for gout.

- **OBESITY:** Being overweight increases the risk of osteoarthritis as well as gout. It is linked with higher levels of inflammation, some of which have been linked to imbalances in the gut microbiome (see page 72).

- **VACCINATION:** Being vaccinated against a wide range of diseases is a valuable health-promoting strategy. However, vaccines work by triggering an immune response. In some individuals prone to gout, a vaccination may provoke a flare-up.

- **HOSPITALIZATION AND/OR SURGERY:** Being hospitalized is stressful in itself. Being in the hospital environment, particularly after major surgeries, involves endless disruptions such as dietary changes and medication adjustments. These can lead to dehydration and changes in kidney function. The addition of new medications (for example, water pills) can affect blood uric acid levels. All of these various stressors can potentially trigger gout.

- **LOWER TEMPERATURES:** Areas of the body with less blood flow (ears, toes, fingers) are often cooler. Their reduced temperature can cause urate to crystallize more readily, triggering a gout attack. This might explain why gout attacks are more frequent in the lower extremities, especially the toes, as well as why tophi deposits often appear around ears and fingers.

- **EXTREME DIETING:** Severely limiting your intake of food (as with fasting and regularly skipping meals) can cause cells to rapidly break down, triggering gout. If you are fasting, your body resorts to breaking down protein as a source of fuel. This massive protein breakdown triggers the release of purines, leading to a rapid increase in uric acid levels.

ENVIRONMENTAL TRIGGERS

It's important to note that abrupt shifts in uric acid blood levels, whether up or down, can potentially trigger a gout flare. Factors such as dehydration and various types of trauma can rapidly change the uric acid levels in the blood.

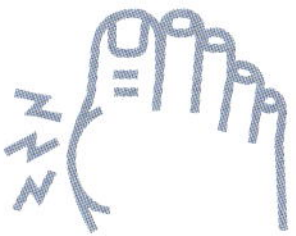

Gout: A Diagnostic Primer

1 **Recognize the Signs and Symptoms of Gout**

- Excruciating pain, frequently affecting the big toe. The area appears red and swollen and feels hot.

- Gout attacks happen more often at night.

2 **Crack the Environmental Code**

- Make sure your doctor takes a detailed medical history. This reveals a lot about a patient. Family history is important, as gout has a genetic component.

- The existence of other conditions such as obesity, high blood sugar, hypertension and/or kidney disease can also signal the possibility of gout.

- Know that some medications can trigger flare-ups.

3 **Use Your Power Tools**

- Have your doctor dive into the pool of available diagnostics, from basic laboratory tests to the most advanced imaging technologies. See page 38, *Lab and Imaging Tests Used to Diagnose Gout.*

CHAPTER 3

Living with Gout

THIS CHAPTER IS full of useful information on living with gout. We further discuss the importance of prevention, and examine how to treat gout both in the short term and the long term.

I believe in a balanced approach. We look at what kinds of medications can be used and when are they appropriate. Understanding that gout is never a stand-alone disease, but rather a disease that can signal other chronic conditions such as high blood pressure, diabetes and obesity, we also see how changing your lifestyle can work with other current treatments for those conditions.

Then we consider the role of food in gout. We dig into why weight matters and why certain foods such as meat, sugars, processed foods and alcoholic beverages can trigger gout attacks. We look at how your gut plays an important role in gout. We review certain diets and learn the benefits of the Mediterranean dietary pattern. Finally, we examine gout-friendly foods (including cherries, vegetables, legumes, whole grains and good sources of protein and fats) and discuss whether certain supplements advertised as good for gout have any scientific basis.

Whether you develop a disease depends more on environmental factors such as diet, physical activity and exposures to toxins than on inherited genetic variants.

Many practitioners are uncertain about when and how to treat gout. As noted, despite being a relatively common condition, gout remains a poorly managed disease. Many patients remain undiagnosed for years. Many others do not receive proper treatment. Both situations set the stage for further complications beyond those directly related to gout. These include diabetes, heart disease and even premature death. I cannot stress too strongly that gout is not just pain and swelling in the big toe. It signals a systemic disease that affects multiple organs.

Prevention Trumps Cure

The best approach to managing any disease is preventing it before
it develops or, failing that, nipping it in the bud as soon as it shows
up. Fortunately, we have numerous tools, from pharmaceuticals to
easy lifestyle modifications, that help us grapple with gout and slow
its progression through the body.

When someone presents with a gout attack, we can consider
various medications that work quickly to relieve pain. There are
also drugs that take longer to act, helping to keep uric acid levels
under control. All have potential risks as well as benefits and should
only be used with expert medical guidance.

Knowing you have a family history of gout gives you some
power over the disease. It tells you that you are vulnerable, likely
because you have genetic variants related to uric acid control.
Clearly, you can't choose your parents. However, you can make
smart and healthy lifestyle choices that will help to keep gout at bay.

Many studies have shown that a healthy lifestyle is the key
determinant in beating back disease and extending your lifespan.
Specifically, eating a nutritious diet, maintaining a normal weight,
being physically active and not smoking or over-imbibing alcohol
significantly reduce your chances of developing chronic diseases.

Thanks to the relatively new science of epigenetics, we are
gaining insight into how genetics and lifestyle are linked. Although
your genes are permanent, they are not static. They react to lifestyle
impacts by changing how they are expressed.

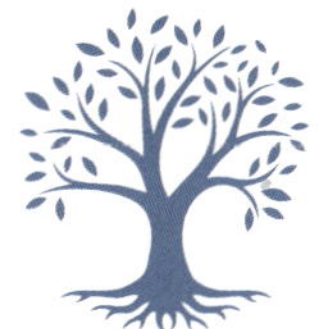

Basically, researchers have found that lifestyle operates hand in
hand with genetic risk. Current research shows that while genes
can raise your risk of developing certain diseases, they are far from
a guarantee that you will succumb to the condition. Whether you
develop a disease depends more on environmental factors such as
diet, physical activity and exposures to toxins than on inherited
genetic variants.

TAKE CONTROL OF YOUR RISK FACTORS

Your genes and your weight are powerful partners. If gout runs in your family,
carrying extra weight might speed up your chances of developing the disease
at a younger age.

However, if you have a family history of gout, making positive lifestyle
changes will mitigate your risk. We may not have control over our genes, but
we do control our daily lives and habits, which inevitably influence our health
and the diseases we develop.

If you have a family history of gout, this finding is very good news. It may not prevent you from developing the disease, but it does alert you, and then you can manage it more effectively. It puts you in the driver's seat when gout is lurking on the sidelines and even if it has already flared up.

This finding applies to other chronic diseases as well, including diabetes and heart disease. Numerous studies have shown that positive lifestyle habits promote healthy patterns of gene expression, helping to keep disease at bay, extending the number of years you remain free of debilitating disease.

Managing Gout

As discussed, there is much uncertainty even within the medical profession about how to manage gout. Practitioners often see treatment as a dilemma. Do they choose to provide short-term relief from pain or initiate longer-term therapy to lower uric acid levels? Do they start long-term treatment during a gout attack or wait until the attack is resolved?

In fact, both approaches are appropriate, depending on the situation. When a patient presents with severe pain during a gout attack, providing relief is paramount. However, once gout is diagnosed, longer-term therapy should be undertaken to keep the condition under control. And yes, you can start long-term treatment during a gout attack.

Short-Term Treatment

A gout attack is agonizing. Relieving that pain is the first thing that any patient is looking to receive and any physician wants to offer. When dealing with a gout attack, the primary objectives are to relieve the pain, reduce inflammation and prevent future episodes.

Relieve the Pain

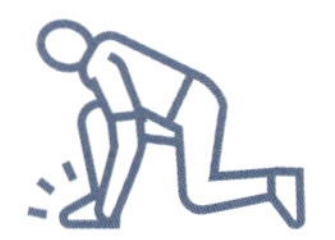

Gout is excruciatingly painful. It is important to alleviate that pain as quickly as possible. That means treatment with an appropriate pain-relieving medication.

Reduce Inflammation

Minimizing inflammation supports pain relief. It also improves joint mobility and helps to limit damage to the joints. Nonsteroidal anti-inflammatory medications (NSAIDs) or steroids are commonly used to achieve this objective.

Prevent Future Episodes

Although the immediate priority is addressing the flare-up, long-term strategies to prevent recurrent attacks should be introduced in order to slow down gout's inevitable progression throughout the body. Once the pain abates, that is the time to discuss longer-term strategies directed at controlling gout. This would include medications to lower uric acid levels and lifestyle modifications.

Medications to Treat a Gout Attack

Basically, medication is the immediate necessary intervention when you have an attack of gout. Once the pain is under control, treatment should shift from pain relief to uric acid control.

Medications that can help during a gout attack include colchicine, NSAIDs and steroids.

GOUT MEDICATIONS		
To relieve gout attacks	**For long-term treatment**	
Colchicine	**Oral therapy**	**IV Therapy**
NSAIDs	Allopurinol	Pegloticase
Prednisone	Febuxostat	

Colchicine

This medication derived from a type of crocus has been used for centuries, effectively reducing the inflammation and pain associated with a gout attack. However, colchicine may have side effects, including nausea, vomiting, abdominal cramping and diarrhea. If you experience any of these, call your doctor.

NOTE: When using colchicine, timing is crucial: Treatment needs to begin within the first 24 hours of an attack. If you have been diagnosed with gout, keep a supply of the medication on hand to ensure that you don't miss this critical window.

Nonsteroidal Anti-Inflammatory Medications (NSAIDs)

If colchicine is not available or the 24-hour window of opportunity was missed, the next best option might be NSAIDs. When experiencing pain, many patients take NSAIDs, as some are available as over-the-counter medications (naproxen, ibuprofen). Others (diclofenac, meloxicam, celecoxib, indomethacin) require a prescription.

Be aware that NSAIDs can have side effects. They may lead to ulcerations in your stomach, gastrointestinal bleeding (indicated by black, dark stools), heart attacks and kidney damage.

CAUTION: Patients with a history of heart or kidney disease should avoid NSAIDs. The excessive use of these medications can lead to heart attacks, heart failure and strokes, as well as kidney failure.

Prednisone

There are situations where neither colchicine or NSAIDs are good options, when patients might have missed the window of opportunity for colchicine or if they have also kidney disease. In these situations, steroid medications such as prednisone (and its derivates) are a great alternative or the next appropriate step.

The most potent anti-inflammatory medications that we have to reduce pain and swelling within hours, or up to a few days, are steroids. Steroids can come in the forms of pills or injections. The most common oral steroid that I use in my practice is prednisone.

However, in some cases, a steroid injection can work wonders. In patients with kidney disease, steroid injections are preferred, since NSAIDs can increase the risk of kidney disfunction. In patients with a knee attack that impairs their walking, an injection provides faster relief, since, unlike a systemic therapy (taking oral prednisone), the therapy is targeted to the specific joint and symptoms of the attack. Also, in patients with diabetes or severe depression or insomnia, oral prednisone can worsen those symptoms, increasing glucose blood levels and worsening depression and insomnia. Not only does an injection work faster, it produces fewer side effects.

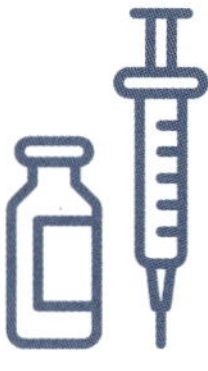

Managing Uric Acid

Consistently high uric acid levels (hyperuricemia) are at the root of gout. As noted, excessive accumulation of uric acid affects many bodily systems, setting the stage for numerous chronic conditions. That is why it's so important to keep uric acid levels under control.

Urate-Lowering Therapy

These days we have several go-to medications for managing gout over the long term. They work by decreasing the uric acid production in the body, specifically by inhibiting an enzyme called xanthine oxidase. These urate-lowering therapy (ULT) medications include allopurinol, febuxostat and pegloticase.

LONG-TERM TREATMENT

It took years for gout to develop, so you shouldn't expect to fix it in a day. To begin with, it will take a long time to bring uric acid levels down even using medication.

Allopurinol

Allopurinol is the most prescribed medication for long-term management of gout. Allopurinol effectively lowers uric acid levels, reducing the frequency of flare-ups and preventing the formation of tophi. It is typically the first-line treatment for gout. After allopurinol is metabolized, it is excreted by the kidneys, so dosage needs to be adjusted for patients with kidney disease. However, a lower dose of the medication is still appropriate for patients with kidney disease. Allopurinol is recommended for:

- People with frequent gout flares

- People with tophi

- People with uric acid kidney stones

- People with chronic kidney disease (dosage adjusted based on kidney function)

SIDE EFFECTS: Allopurinol is generally well tolerated but, like any medication, it can cause side effects. These include skin rash, nausea, diarrhea and increased liver enzymes. Severe allergic reactions such as Stevens-Johnson syndrome (a rash that can extend and cause blisters of the skin and mucosae) are rare but require immediate medical attention. If you experience unusual symptoms while taking allopurinol, consult your doctor promptly.

Febuxostat

Like allopurinol, febuxostat lowers uric acid levels by inhibiting xanthine oxidase. Febuxostat is recommended for:

- People who cannot tolerate or have contraindications to allopurinol, or those who can't get uric acid levels down using allopurinol

- People with frequent gout flares

- People with tophi

- People with uric acid kidney stones

- People with chronic kidney disease (dosage adjusted)

SIDE EFFECTS: Febuxostat is generally well tolerated. It has been associated with elevated liver enzymes, nausea, joint pain and skin rash. Severe allergic reactions and cardiovascular events are rare but require immediate medical attention.

CAUTION: Febuxostat should be avoided if you have a history of heart attacks or other cardiovascular problems, as it has been linked with an increased risk of cardiovascular events.

Pegloticase

If neither allopurinol or febuxostat is successful in decreasing blood uric acid levels at up-to-maximum doses, this newer infusion (intravenous therapy) drug is available. Pegloticase is used alone and not in combination with any other urate-lowering therapy.

When using this medication, patients will need to check their uric acid levels before and after each infusion as part of the infusion protocol. If their uric acid blood level remains persistently greater than 6 mg/dL, that is a sign that it has lost its efficacy and the medication must be discontinued. Pegloticase is recommended for:

- Patients with recurrent episodes of gout and tophi

- Those for whom other uric acid–lowering medications have not been effective

SIDE EFFECTS: The side effects associated with pegloticase can be dangerous. The infusion is given in a hospital setting to allow for patients to be monitored during the process. Potential side effects include anaphylaxis and other infusion reactions during and after the infusion. To prevent potential reactions to the infusion, researchers paired a weekly dose of methotrexate (an immunosuppressive medication) with pegloticase infusions. This seemed to decrease the incidence of allergic reactions and improved the treatment response to pegloticase. See the box, below, about other potential problems.

CAUTION: Pegloticase has been pulled out of the market by the manufacturer in the European Union. While it is still FDA approved in the United States, it is seen as a last resort.

SPEEDY RESULTS BUT POTENTIAL PROBLEMS

While it might take many months, even years, for oral medications to significantly improve a patient's condition, pegloticase has the potential to achieve similar results in just a few months. However, the drug is something of a last resort for severe gout patients, for a number of reasons, including:

- It is an infusion, which means it is administered intravenously. Visits to a clinic every two weeks are very inconvenient for many patients.
- It is very expensive. Insurance companies will not approve its use unless patients fail therapy with allopurinol and febuxostat.
- It can cause severe allergic reactions.
- It often doesn't work. The success rate in reducing uric acid levels and tophi is only 40%.

Lifestyle Versus Medication: It's Not Either/Or

Obviously, I am not against using medication to treat gout. It is a regular part of my practice. However, as I tell my patients, medication can be a double-edged sword. You can benefit from it, but it will likely come with side effects, some more severe for certain individuals. It can also be very costly to take medication for what will likely be years.

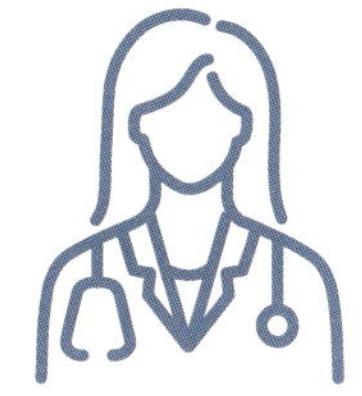

In North America our medical system leans heavily toward treating gout solely with medication. There are many reasons for this. You might be surprised to learn, for instance, that most doctors know very little about nutrition; medical school usually provides only four to six hours of nutritional education over the course of 10 years of training. Yet awareness of nutrition is vital to maintaining a healthy lifestyle.

Moreover, pharmaceutical companies spent vast amounts of money marketing their products directly to doctors, who are inundated with information on their benefits. And much of the research into treating disease is at least partially funded by the private sector. Drug companies have the deep pockets needed to conduct extensive studies.

Another problem is nutritional research itself. Funding is a problem because there is no patented product that can be sold at the end of a potentially costly process. Most studies are small, spotlighting the benefits of specific nutrients when treating a particular disease.

The truth is, nutrition studies are hard to control due to their numerous variables. Unfortunately, many studies focusing on the effect of specific nutrients have not shown that individual nutrients significantly impact chronic disease. The problem with this approach is that we do not eat specific nutrients. We eat food containing those nutrients.

Instead of trying to treat any disease with a specific nutrient, we should consider the array of nutrients provided by the food we eat, and address the disease with the right quality and quantity of food.

We do not eat specific nutrients.
We eat food containing those nutrients,

Medications work by targeting specific bodily systems. But so do nutrients from our food. A healthier lifestyle that includes healthy eating will translate into using less medication, which reduces the risk of side effects.

The *American College of Rheumatology Gout Guideline,* updated by experts in the field in 2020, acknowledges that nutrition plays a role in gout attacks. However, it fails to emphasize its potential value in managing the condition, noting the small size or limited duration of relevant studies. Patients are often open to approaches involving lifestyle modifications, particularly regarding healthy eating, but at the moment their physicians are hesitant or not sufficiently educated in the nutrition field to provide them with information on dietary interventions.

For decades, the medical community has been actively debating the role that nutrition can play in managing gout. However, at least one connection isn't debatable: gout cases have risen dramatically over the past decades. Today there are 53 million people diagnosed with gout worldwide. That increase parallels our increased consumption of ultraprocessed foods. The encouraging news is that over the past few years, I've noticed more and more physicians taking an interest in nutrition and how it can help with managing chronic disease.

A BALANCED APPROACH

I think of my own approach as balanced. It combines the disease-fighting benefits of a healthy lifestyle with accepted medical therapies. I feel strongly that any treatment protocol for gout should begin by identifying where lifestyle changes will be helpful.

It likely took a couple of decades for your uric acid levels to rise to the point where they trigger a gout attack. It will take longer than just few months of dietary changes to bring those numbers down to a manageable level.

Another thing to consider is that treating gout on its own might not be enough to change your health outcome. You also need to control your weight, blood pressure, blood sugar and cholesterol to increase your lifespan.

Today there are 53 million people diagnosed with gout worldwide.

Gout and Other Chronic Conditions

Gout is not a stand-alone disease. I can't stress too strongly that gout is not an isolated condition. As noted earlier, gout almost never appears alone. It is considered a metabolic disease and is usually linked with conditions associated with metabolic syndrome. Most patients suffering from gout have other chronic conditions such as hypertension (high blood pressure), diabetes, psoriasis and/or obesity. Some of these diseases are strongly linked to an increased incidence of gout. A common denominator of hypertension, insulin resistance, obesity and psoriasis is chronic ongoing inflammation.

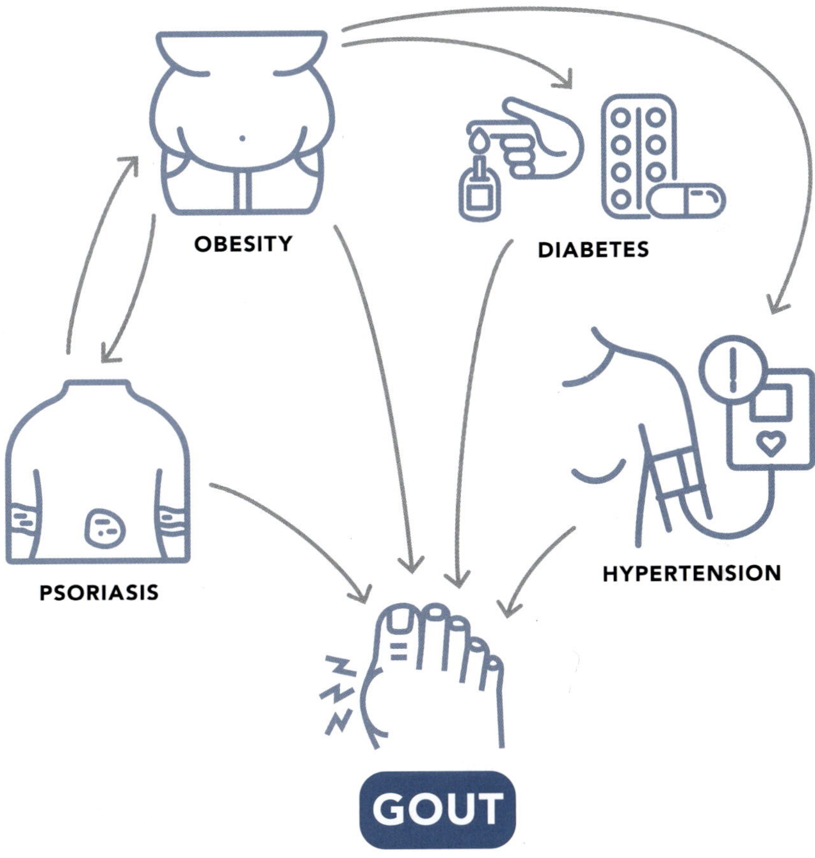

Gout and other chronic conditions. Most patients suffering from gout have other chronic conditions such as hypertension, diabetes, psoriasis and/or obesity.

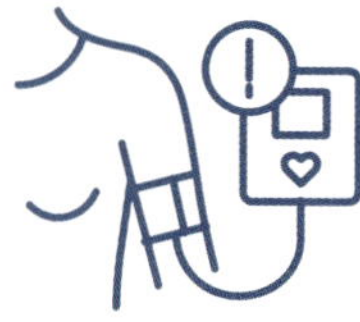

Hypertension

People suffering from high blood pressure will have decreased blood flow to the kidneys, reducing the excretion of uric acid. This will lead to increased levels of uric acid in the blood.

Moreover, they are often prescribed diuretics (water pills), which help to lower blood pressure by increasing the salt and water excreted in urine, thereby decreasing blood volume and blood pressure. Some diuretics can increase uric acid levels by reducing excretion from the kidneys, raising gout risk. Other antihypertensive medications (captopril, lisinopril) may increase the risk of developing gout. These medications are, however, generally safe to use under medical supervision.

Diabetes and Obesity

These conditions are closely connected. Obesity leads to insulin resistance (your cells become less responsive to the hormone insulin, which is essential in regulating blood sugar), a common precursor to diabetes. In addition, obesity is clearly associated with more inflammation. Fat cells produce substances that induce inflammation. Inflammation increases the likelihood of developing gout.

Obesity, Psoriasis and Gout

Like obesity, psoriasis, an autoimmune disease characterized by red, scaly patches on the skin, has close links with gout. Excessive adipose tissue increases the production of certain molecules (adipokines) that spark inflammation. Thus, excessive inflammation will worsen psoriasis. Many people with psoriasis need to control their weight because it helps to control their skin disease.

Psoriasis and Gout

In some cases, people with psoriasis also develop a painful joint condition called psoriatic arthritis, which shares many symptoms with gout (see page 24). However, many people with psoriasis can also develop gout as a secondary diagnosis. Making the distinction between psoriatic arthritis and gout can be quite challenging.

Weight Matters

Being overweight is extremely problematic for your health. Obese people are likely to have a shorter lifespan than those with a healthy weight. They are also at higher risk for many chronic conditions, including hypertension, insulin resistance (a major risk factor for type 2 diabetes) and heart disease. Unsurprisingly, they are also more likely to develop osteoarthritis and/or gout.

Body mass index (BMI) is a measure of how much fat someone has in relation to their height. Although it is not a perfect diagnostic tool, a high BMI is a useful predictor of potential health problems. Weight gain and obesity increase the risk of developing gout at an early age, especially if you have the disease in your family.

It doesn't take much extra weight, particularly if it collects around your middle, to sabotage your health. For instance, one study published in the journal *Cell Systems* in 2018 found that even a slight weight gain (6 pounds/2.7 kg) negatively affected the subjects' immune system and their microbiome while increasing inflammation throughout the body.

An Ideal Body Weight

One of the most valuable lifestyle changes a person with gout can make is achieving and maintaining an ideal body weight. If you gain a lot of weight, the risk of developing gout increases significantly. Moreover, the disease may show up at a younger age.

Research clearly links a healthy weight with helping to keep gout under control. One prospective study, which followed 47,000 men for 12 years, showed that weight loss decreased the risk of developing gout. Men who gained approximately 29 pounds or more (more than 13 kg) were twice as likely to develop gout compared to those who maintained their weight. In contrast, weight loss of more than 10 pounds (4.5 kg) was associated with a reduced risk of developing gout.

One systematic review of multiple studies (published in 2017) showed that when overweight and obese individuals with gout lost weight, their gout attacks became less frequent over the long term because their uric acid levels declined.

A *prospective study* is a type of study that follows a group of participants and observe if they develop a disease over a certain period of time. The study focuses on identifying factors that increase or decrease the risk of that disease. At the beginning of the study, none of the participants have the disease of interest.

GRADUAL WEIGHT LOSS WORKS BEST

If you are worried about gout, it's not a good idea to diet aggressively. Eating very little (to the point of starving the body of nutrition) and dehydration can trigger gout attacks. A gradual weight loss of 3 to 5 pounds (1 to 2 kg) monthly is recommended.

Bariatric Surgery

Many people with gout are also obese. In such cases, a procedure called bariatric surgery might be an effective way to achieve significant weight loss. This surgery has also been shown to decrease the incidence of or improve associated medical conditions such as diabetes, high blood pressure and even heart disease.

One Swedish study of obese patients who had no diagnosis of gout and underwent bariatric surgery showed that their uric acid level decreased significantly, reducing the risk of developing gout; these patients were followed for a period of 19 years after the surgery.

Bariatric surgery also seems to be beneficial in obese patients already suffering from gout, even though in the month immediately following the surgery, these patients may have more gout attacks than usual. However, about a year after their surgery, the incidence of their attacks should decrease significantly. There is some evidence that weight loss resulting from bariatric surgery might have a beneficial impact on the gut microbiota. It appears to increase bacterial diversity, boosting the incidence of species that help to tame inflammation and lower uric acid production.

Research shows that uric acid levels begin to decrease as early as three months following bariatric surgery, and that these lower levels were maintained for at least three years.

CASE STUDY — ROBERT

Robert is a 58-year-old man who has been battling gout, high blood pressure, diabetes and obesity for many years. His health recently took a significant turn for the worse when he had a heart attack. With a BMI of 40, Robert was severely obese, which complicated his health problems.

His heart attack served as a wake-up call, motivating Robert to improve his health. As part of his new health regimen, he decided to undergo bariatric surgery, a decision he made after careful consultation with his physician. He understood that the surgery would not only help him lose weight but also improve his blood pressure and diabetes, both of which were closely linked with obesity.

The first month following his surgery was challenging. Robert experienced four gout attacks. However, nine months after surgery, his health showed marked improvement. His serum urate levels had reduced significantly, from a high 13mg/dL before surgery to 8mg/dL, and his gout attacks reduced to just one in the nine months following the surgery.

Moreover, his other health conditions started to improve. His BMI reached 30, his blood pressure readings stabilized and his diabetes was better managed.

Bariatric Surgery Delivers Many Benefits

My patient Robert's high blood pressure and diabetes improved after his surgery. When you lose weight, insulin resistance improves, so diabetes is better controlled, and blood pressure decreases because kidney function improves.

Regular Physical Activity

In addition to strengthening muscles and improving insulin resistance and cardiovascular function, regular exercise supports maintaining a healthy weight, which helps with managing gout. It is also well documented that regular physical activity helps to control inflammation. One 2020 study that recruited 30 gout patients and followed them for a year found that those who were physically active had lower levels of C-reactive protein (a measure of inflammation) and significantly fewer flare-ups, and experienced much less pain than those who were more sedentary.

Battling Flare-Ups

Gout attacks can be triggered by many different factors. We call these "triggers." Some are not under your control, while others are manageable. Think about being admitted to hospital or being prescribed a medication that causes your uric acid levels to rise. These are triggers that are not within your control. (See *Chapter 2: Diagnosing Gout* for more information regarding gout triggers, including some unexpected triggers on page 45.) However, taking charge of your lifestyle, consuming certain foods and drinking certain beverages is something you can control.

Food and Beverage Triggers for Gout

Certain foods and beverages have a well-established link with gout attacks. These include:

- Red meat, processed meats, organ meats and shellfish

- Some beverages, including beer, protein shakes, spirits and liquor

- Some canned foods

- Instant foods and sugary treats

- Ultraprocessed foods including packaged snacks, baked goods, and some sweetened breakfast cereals

ULTRAPROCESSED FOODS

These manufactured edibles are formulations of unhealthy fats, excessive sugar and salt and other substances, carefully calibrated to whet your appetite for more. Research shows that replacing just 20% of these foods with unprocessed options can significantly reduce the risk of gout.

Red Meat

Red meats include beef, pork, lamb, veal, game meats, and offal (animal organs and entrails such as liver and kidneys). This category also includes processed meats.

These meats are problematic for people with gout because they are rich in purines (see pages 31–32). Consuming large quantities can increase uric acid levels in the blood.

THE SOURCE OF PROTEIN MATTERS

Many people consume meat because they believe it is the best source of high-quality protein, which plays a pivotal role in maintaining health. However, when our bodies break down proteins, purines are produced. As noted, foods that are high in purines have been shown to increase the risk of recurrent gout attacks.

However, when it comes to gout, all proteins aren't created equal. For instance, one large national U.S. survey showed that the impact of protein intake depends on the source of protein. Unlike meat-related protein, the protein from dairy or legumes was associated with lower uric acid levels.

Shellfish

Shellfish is considered seafood. Not all seafood is bad for people with gout, but if you have gout, shellfish consumption can raise uric acid levels, triggering a gout attack. Shellfish such as shrimp, crab, lobster, mussels, clams and oysters are high in purines, but low in omega-3 fatty acids, which have an anti-inflammatory effect that helps to balance their purine content. To read about seafood that does contain omega-3s, see page 84.

High-Fructose Corn Syrup

High-fructose corn syrup (HFCS) is a manufactured sweetener found in many foods and drinks, primarily packaged baked goods, soft drinks and energy drinks. Products containing HFCS are usually ultraprocessed foods that also contain unhealthy fats and large quantities of salt. In addition, these foods provide very little fiber and other nutrients. Excessive consumption of foods and/ or beverages containing HFCS will cause fructose to build up in your body. As fructose gets metabolized through liver, an excessive amount will eventually lead to non-alcoholic fatty liver disease.

Consuming fructose in HFCS is very different from eating fruits that are high in fructose. Fruit also provides fiber and other nutrients, which slows down fructose metabolism. Eating fruit regularly does not cause non-alcoholic fatty liver disease.

HFCS has been shown to raise uric acid levels in your body in two ways, through your liver and your kidneys:

- In processing HFCS, your liver generates substances that are converted into uric acid.

- HFCS reduces the amount of uric acid your kidneys expel, while boosting its reabsorption in your body, elevating levels in your blood.

Excessive HFCS consumption has also been linked to insulin resistance, which will lead to diabetes. When the body becomes less responsive to insulin, it raises insulin levels in the blood, triggering the production of uric acid.

High consumption of HFCS has also been associated with obesity and metabolic syndrome (see page 26), both of which are recognized risk factors for gout.

Glucose and Fructose Versus HFCS

When many people think about sugar they imagine "glucose." However, commercial sugar is a combination of glucose and fructose. Both are absorbed through the intestine but they are metabolized differently. Glucose can potentially be metabolized by your body's cells with the help of the hormone insulin. It is transformed into energy at the cellular level.

When we refer to an increase in blood sugar, we refer to excess glucose in the blood. Excessive glucose can be deposited in the body in the form of fats, leading to increased weight.

Fructose, on the other hand, is metabolized through the liver. It does not need insulin. However, excessive amounts of fructose can lead to fat, which can be deposited in the liver, causing fatty liver disease (non-alcoholic fatty liver disease). Too much fructose may also lead to excessive amounts of uric acid, increasing the risk of gout.

As noted, fructose from fruits comes along with many other nutrients, including fiber, which support your metabolism, decreasing the risk of gout. On the other hand, high-fructose corn syrup just provides excessive amounts of fructose.

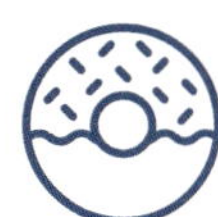

IS THE FRUCTOSE IN FRUIT BAD FOR ME?

The fructose in HFCS is a manufactured product. It contains much higher levels of fructose than found in any fruit, making it more difficult for your body to process. However, when found naturally in fruit, where it resides with other nutrients, including fiber, fructose is a healthy source of energy.

Sugar-Sweetened Beverages

Sodas and sugar-sweetened juices, including many supposedly "healthy" juices, are linked to an increased risk of gout attacks; The added sugar (mostly in the form of HFCS) provides empty calories, while the lack of fiber will raise the blood sugar levels and contributes to increased uric acid production.

Protein Shakes

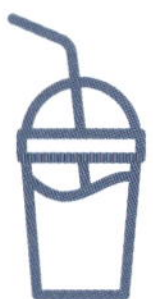

Protein shakes are very popular for people trying to lose weight or building muscle through exercise. These drinks promise to be a quick fix by providing more protein in a box or can. They are made with protein powders obtained from plants, whey (concentrate and isolate) and casein. However, despite their promises, they raise the risk for a gout attack because they contain excessive amounts of protein and also sugar (in the form of HFCS).

The average daily amount of protein recommended is 45 grams for females and 55 grams for men. Considering that most shake powders contain about 25 to 30 grams of protein per scoop, consuming these beverages in excess leads to high purine production and a rapid increase of the uric acid in the blood.

Moreover, a recent report from a nonprofit organization called the Clean Label Project screened about 130 products that qualified as "protein shakes." These researchers identified 130 types of toxins, including many heavy metals such as lead, arsenic and mercury. Some of these substances are linked to cancer.

COFFEE: KEEP IT BLACK

Coffee is the magical potion many of us rely on to bring our brains back to life when we wake up in the morning. The problem is, if you add copious amounts of sugar and cream, you are adding HFCS and unhealthy fats to your favorite morning pick-me-up, thereby increasing your risk of developing gout.

On the other hand, if your taste leans toward a steaming cup of unadulterated black coffee, you might be helping to keep gout at bay. A study of more than 40,000 men followed over about 12 years showed that long-term black coffee consumption, especially if decaffeinated, reduced their risk of developing gout.

Another study, spanning over 20 years, showed that drinking more than four cups of coffee a day can slightly lower uric acid levels in the blood. These findings were not seen in people drinking tea.

So far, we do not have any clinical trials regarding the use of coffee in people with gout.

While I typically don't advise patients to consume four cups of coffee daily, especially those with high blood pressure or kidney issues, when asked about coffee in relation to gout, I advise that a single cup of black coffee in the morning may be beneficial. Remember, moderation is essential.

Alcoholic Beverages

Drinking alcohol is a potent trigger for gout. Not only does it increase uric acid production, but it may also inhibit its excretion.

Understanding how alcohol, especially the type of alcohol you consume, can affect your risk of developing gout attacks is an important step in managing the condition. If you have a diagnosis of gout, drinking alcohol may set the stage for more gout attacks. That is valid for all types of alcohol from beer to liquor and, in some cases, even moderate amounts of wine. The following beverages can be troublesome for people with gout. They are listed in order of their potentially harmful effects.

Beer

Many studies show a clear connection between beer consumption and gout risk. One study that followed 47,000 men without a diagnosis of gout over the course of 12 years linked alcohol intake in general with an increased risk of gout. Beer was the worst perpetrator.

Consuming two or more beers per day has been found to double the likelihood of developing your first gout attack, compared to people who didn't drink beer.

BEER: A DOUBLE WHAMMY

As an alcoholic beverage, beer has been shown to slow down uric acid excretion by the kidneys, thus further raising blood levels of the substance. In addition, beer contains brewer's yeast, which is rich in purines, leading to increase uric acid production in your body.

Spirits

Spirits such as whiskey and vodka can also contribute to gout.
Despite posing a slightly lower risk than beer, spirits have a high
alcohol content that can disrupt uric acid elimination, setting the
stage for a gout attack. Men who drink liquor have been shown
to have a 1.6-fold increased risk of developing gout.

Heavy and prolonged alcohol consumption, particularly
of distilled liquor, could lead to the development of chronic
tophaceous gout (the severe form of the condition characterized
by the formation of tophi). One study in people with gout linked
quantity, frequency and duration of consumption (based on weekly
intake and a history of drinking alcohol for more than 10 years)
with tophi development.

Wine

When it comes to wine, there is a difference between people with
a predisposition to developing gout versus people who have already
been diagnosed with the disease.

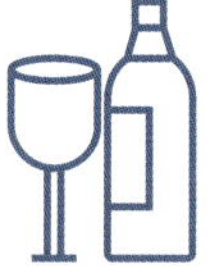

In people without a diagnosis of gout, research suggests that
moderate wine intake might protect against developing the disease.
One study showed that drinking two 4-ounce (120 mL) glasses
of wine per day was not associated with an increased risk of
developing gout.

However, this does not give wine lovers free rein to drink
excessively. Often studies view wine consumption within a broader
context. In general terms, some wine enthusiasts are likely to
adhere to a healthier lifestyle, including eating a nutritious diet and
exercising regularly.

For those with an existing gout diagnosis, sometimes moderate
wine consumption can pose a risk. One study showed that drinking
more than two 5-ounce glasses of wine per day has been linked to
an increased risk of gout flare-ups.

Although drinking wine may also still be beneficial for many
other health reasons, I do advise my patients who have gout under
control, meaning that their uric acid level is consistently within the
target range (<6.5 mg/dL) and they are taking their medications,
to drink wine only rarely, limiting it to one glass once or twice
a week. As shown in the *Gout Food Pyramid* (see page 85), wine
consumption in people with gout should be limited to rarely.

Watch the Combinations

While individual foods can be triggers, certain combinations of foods and/or food and beverages magnify their potentially negative effects. In these situations, the quantity consumed also has an impact on whether a gout flare-up will result.

For example, drinking beer and eating foods high in purines such as red meat and shellfish can amplify the risk of a gout flare-up.

Combinations to Avoid If You Have Gout

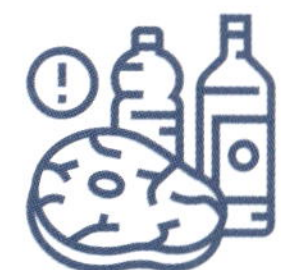

- **BEER AND SHRIMP:** The high purine content in both can cause uric acid levels to surge, leading to a potential flare-up.

- **WINE AND STEAK:** The purines in red meat combined with moderate to excessive alcohol consumption can trigger gout.

- **PANCAKES IN SWEETENED SYRUP, WASHED DOWN WITH SODA:** Both manufactured syrups and soda are loaded with high-fructose corn syrup (see page 62).

- **FRIED FOODS WITH BEER:** This classic combination of unhealthy fats and high-purine beer is a recipe for a painful gout episode.

- **FEASTING:** Gorging, as you might be inclined to do at a special occasion meal, can overburden the body's ability to process uric acid, resulting in a gout attack.

Dietary Approaches to Managing Gout

When managing gout, foods to avoid are only half the story. The foods you eat can be equally helpful in preventing flare-ups or even in preventing gout from developing in the first place. Later in this chapter you will find the *Gout Food Pyramid,* which I designed to summarize the food choices you should make when suffering from gout (see page 85). First, however, let's look at some of the various dietary approaches to managing gout and the science behind those approaches.

CASE STUDY   **JULIA**

Julia was a 64-year-old woman without any significant health complications. She enjoyed a typical Western-style diet—lots of red meat, fried foods and sugary snacks—and drank two glasses of beer every night with dinner. Like many individuals, Julia didn't think twice about her dietary choices. After all, she had managed to maintain a reasonable weight, and her energy levels were good for her moderately active lifestyle.

However, as Julia entered menopause, her situation started to change. Her energy levels took a significant hit and she gained about 20 pounds (almost 10 kg). This was a new experience for her. Not only did she feel uncomfortable in her body, but she started to have gout attacks.

In the beginning, she had one every year; two years ago, the frequency increased to one every other month. She noticed small, white, hard bumps on her fingers that were sometimes painful. Her fingers and toes started to change in appearance. Julia's father had suffered from gout, but she didn't think she was vulnerable because the condition is less common in women.

The attacks were excruciating and hindered her ability to work or spend time with her family. Testing revealed a high uric acid level of 10 mg/dL. Julia started treatment with allopurinol but continued to have gout attacks. Consequently, she wanted to explore additional ways to combat her condition. She decided to drastically change her diet, transitioning from a typical Western-style diet to what's known as the Mediterranean diet. She significantly increased her intake of fruits, vegetables, whole grains and lean proteins such as fish, while reducing her consumption of red meat, processed foods and added sugars. Every day, she took a 45-minute walk.

After six months of adhering to her new diet, Julia got her uric acid levels rechecked. They had decreased only slightly, to 9 mg/dL, which was initially disheartening. However, she noticed a dramatic change in the frequency of her gout attacks, which reduced to about one attack a year. Moreover, her energy was high, and she had lost about 10 pounds (4.5 kg).

The Western-Style Diet

The Western-style diet (also called the Standard American Diet, or SAD) is a term used to describe typical eating habits that incorporate a lot of prepackaged foods, refined grains, fried foods, processed meats, conventionally raised animal products, red meat, high-sugar drinks, candies and other sweets. Increasingly, scientists are recognizing the connection between a Western-style diet, alcohol consumption and heightened uric acid levels. For those with a family history of gout, dietary shifts can be vital in helping to keep the disease at bay or delay its onset at a younger age.

The Mediterranean Dietary Pattern

The so-called "Mediterranean diet" is an approach to healthy eating built around nutritious whole foods. It a pattern of eating, not a diet. That means it is adaptable to a wide range of food preferences and cultural customs. Basically, it is a plant-forward eating plan, built around natural whole foods such as whole grains, fruits, vegetables, legumes, nuts and seeds, plus healthy fats obtained mainly from fish and olive oil. Red meat, sugar, dairy and eggs are consumed in moderation.

The Mediterranean dietary pattern has been extensively studied and shown to have numerous health benefits, from reducing the risk of heart disease and certain types of cancer to staving off depression. It is consistently recognized by various health organizations as the healthiest eating pattern overall. It also has specific benefits for people with or at risk for gout. These include:

- Lower inflammation. Numerous studies have linked a Mediterranean-style diet to lower inflammation.

- Lower risk of metabolic diseases associated with gout, including high blood pressure, diabetes, and cardiovascular disease

- Less likelihood of developing psoriasis

- Fewer gout flare-ups, likely due to high fiber content, which links to a healthy microbiome

- Lower uric acid levels and lower probability of developing hyperuricemia

A VERY ADAPTABLE EATING PATTERN

Any pattern of eating that includes plenty of plant foods as well as regular consumption of fish and seafood provides the benefits of the Mediterranean diet. Good examples are chicken and vegetable stir-fry on soba noodles, or trout, quinoa, and rapini with pine nuts drizzled with olive oil, or vegetarian tacos with corn tortillas. The key is minimally processed whole ingredients.

The Mediterranean Diet Is Rich in Antioxidants

A Mediterranean-style diet, rich in vegetables, fruits, whole grains, nuts and olive oil, ensures a high intake of nutrients, including vitamins B, C, E and folate, as well as many minerals and phytonutrients, including beta-carotene and polyphenols. All of these nutrients have been shown to have antioxidant effects, which means they fight disease-promoting free radicals, helping to keep oxidative stress under control.

Some studies specifically evaluated the total antioxidant effect of the Mediterranean-style diet. They showed an increase in antioxidant levels across the board (ATTICA study). They also showed a significant impact on how the body metabolizes fats, decreasing bad cholesterol, while increasing good cholesterol (PREDIMED study). When compared to supplements, the Mediterranean diet was shown to be a better approach, most likely because of the combined effects of the multiple antioxidants provided by the various foods.

Oxidative Stress and Gout

When your body produces too many free radicals, oxidative stress results. This imbalance is very bad for your health, potentially causing disease-inducing damage. Certainly, it is a factor in chronic kidney disease, which results when too much uric acid is produced thanks to inflammation and oxidative stress. Eventually, excess uric acid will permeate your cells, where it acts as a pro-oxidant, creating oxidative stress. Some studies, most in animals, suggest that the use of certain antioxidant supplements such as vitamins E and C or combinations of them, and plant-derived polyphenols, including curcumin, flavonoids or probiotics, can reduce oxidative stress.

Although research is still in the emergent stage, it does suggest antioxidants might be a valuable addition to current gout therapy. And the Mediterranean-style diet is abundant in antioxidants.

The DASH Diet

The American Heart Association developed a diet specifically designed to address the needs of people with high blood pressure (hypertension). It is called the DASH (Dietary Approaches to Stop Hypertension) diet. Like the Mediterranean diet, DASH emphasizes the consumption of fruits, vegetables, whole grains and low-fat dairy products while limiting the consumption of red meats, sweets and saturated fats.

One difference between the two dietary approaches is that the DASH diet stresses the need to limit salt (sodium) intake, while emphasizing foods high in potassium, including leafy greens and starchy vegetables such as potatoes and squash.

Clinical studies have demonstrated that people adopting the DASH diet can substantially reduce their blood pressure.

Seventy-four percent of people with gout suffer from hypertension and half of people with hypertension have an increased level of uric acid. Adopting the DASH diet seems to be helpful for people with gout, as it has been shown to directly decrease blood levels of uric acid, especially in people with high values, thus reducing their risk for gout.

The Low-Purine Diet

The low-purine diet was initially discussed when gout was approached from a very specific perspective. This diet tends to focus on avoiding foods that are rich in purines (fish, sardines, shellfish, organ meats, alcohol) while replacing them with fruits, vegetables and whole grains.

One problem with the low-purine approach is that the food choices are so limited, it risks nutritional deficiency. Moreover, eating such a small number of foods on an ongoing basis is challenging because boredom is likely to set in. This makes it more difficult to stick to the diet. Also, it may take years to sufficiently decrease uric acid levels, which means that maintaining such a restrictive diet is not sustainable.

It's also worth noting that science does not support following the low-purine diet to control gout. Basically, there is much more to treating gout than reducing consumption of animal proteins. Other factors such as maintaining a healthy weight, improving insulin resistance and keeping blood pressure under control also play an important role in managing gout.

The Microbiome

Your body hosts countless microbes, but those residing in your gut have the greatest influence on your health. This is known as your gut microbiome. Numerous studies have demonstrated that the bacteria residing in your gut play an essential role in your health because they regulate your metabolism, endocrine and immune systems, among other benefits. In recent years, more and more studies have shown that your gut bacteria influence the onset and progression of gout.

Research suggests that people with gout harbor different species of gut bacteria than people who don't have the disease. That makes the gut microbiota (the living microorganisms, or bacteria, in the microbiome) a potential target in treating gout.

Gut Bacteria and Uric Acid

Studies show that certain species of bacteria in the gut can influence uric acid metabolism. The following are a few examples.

- People with gout have an abundance of certain bacteria such as *Escherichia, Shigella, Fusobacterium* and *Bacteroides,* which increase the production of uric acid at the gut level.

- Fructose is metabolized by gut bacteria. In people with gout, some bacterial species do a poor job of metabolizing fructose, increasing the uric acid production.

- People with gout have fewer species of bacteria that degrade purines and uric acid at the gut level, as well as fewer bacteria that can produce substance that tamp down inflammation.

- People supplementing with probiotics containing bacteria belonging to the *Lactobacillus* family (which have been shown to inhibit the production of uric acid) have lower levels of uric acid in their blood.

As a result of these studies, therapies that target the gut microbiome have drawn significant interest in treating gout, but they are still far from becoming reality.

Fiber: Superfood for Your Gut

Among its benefits, fiber is a primary food source for the bacteria residing in your gut. Studies show that the more fiber you consume, the more robust your microbiome and ultimately the better your health. Increasing your consumption of fiber quickly boosts the types of bacteria residing in your gut. One study showed that eating a high-fiber diet for as little as two weeks spiked bacterial diversity, a marker of gut health.

Don't Forget Polyphenols

Polyphenols are compounds found in plants. Research has shown that polyphenols have antioxidant and anti-inflammatory effects, offering protection against aging, cancer and diabetes. One 2017 study showed that the use of apple polyphenols in overweight people with gout being treated with allopurinol significantly reduced their blood levels of uric acid when compared to people who were treated with medication alone.

Researchers initially believed that fiber was responsible for most of the benefits associated with a healthy microbiome. However, recent research suggests that other substances, especially polyphenols, a type of phytonutrient found in plant foods, are particularly effective at promoting the growth of beneficial bacteria. Unhealthy dietary patterns such as the Western-style diet, which is low in plant foods and dietary fiber, have been shown to undermine your body's ability to metabolize polyphenols.

Flavonoids

Flavonoids are a type of polyphenol. These natural substances are primarily found in fruits, vegetables, tea, grains, legumes, nuts and wine. They are recognized for their antioxidant, anti-inflammatory and cancer-fighting effects. Data from animal studies suggests that supplementation with flavonoids (for example, quercentin) can decrease levels of uric acid by increasing its excretion in urine or by reducing uric acid production in the first place.

YOUR GUT LOVES PLANT FOODS

Research from the American Gut Project has shown that the best way to boost microbial diversity is to eat 30 different plant foods every week.

Probiotics: A Natural Ally

As noted, bacterial diversity is associated with gut health. Over the past century, for numerous reasons, the diversity of bacterial species in our gut has alarmingly diminished. This loss of microbial diversity has correlated with a surge in chronic diseases such as high blood pressure, obesity, diabetes, autoimmune disorders and elevated blood uric acid levels.

Probiotics are live "friendly" or "good" bacteria that have shown promise in promoting gut health. Unsurprisingly, these helpful bacteria are now under the scientific lens, especially in conditions such as hyperuricemia.

Can Probiotics Treat Gout?

Research suggests that certain probiotics (for example, *Lactobacillus brevis* and *Lactobacillus paracasei*) can reduce hyperuricemia through various mechanisms that may affect uric acid production or enhance uric acid excretion. Probiotics have also a direct anti-inflammatory effect and boost the immune system. Although this research is still in early stages, some studies suggest that probiotics have a potential role in managing high uric acid levels.

An analysis of 34 randomized controlled trials that evaluated probiotics' efficacy for various autoimmune diseases, included hyperuricemia and gout. Results from four such trials involving 294 participants indicated that probiotic intervention could improve serum uric acid levels in hyperuricemia and gout patients. Importantly, probiotics did not increase the risk of adverse events across all conditions studied, suggesting they are safe to use.

While these insights are promising, it's important to recognize that this research is still in the early stages. The gut's relationship with hyperuricemia and gout is intricate. While probiotics seem to offer a potential therapeutic avenue, further research needs to confirm these preliminary data.

Gout-Fighting Foods

Although certain foods can trigger gout, there are also some foods that can help to prevent the disease. Nutritional science is moving quickly these days. Through large epidemiologic studies, research is confirming not only that good nutrition works to prevent disease, but also that it works its magic by targeting specific bodily processes.

Fruits, Vegetables and Other Plant Foods

I do not promote a strict vegetarian diet. However, all nutrition experts will tell you that in general North Americans need to boost their consumption of plant foods. I believe in the benefits of a diet that incorporates more plants and less meat. Plant foods provide many of the nutrients you need. This includes vitamins (with the exception of vitamin B12), minerals, fiber and beneficial phytonutrients such as polyphenols and antioxidants.

Consider one Taiwanese study involving about 14,000 participants. These researchers found that lacto-ovo vegetarians (those who also consume dairy and eggs) had the lowest uric acid levels of those studied. They speculated that avoiding purine-rich meat and seafood, in conjunction with consuming more phytochemical-rich plant foods, may limit the production of uric acid while facilitating its excretion. They also noted that vegetarian diets are associated with lower inflammation. One reason is that their high fiber content supports the production of anti-inflammatory substances produced by beneficial gut bacteria.

Importantly, vegetarians were found to have a lower risk of developing gout, even when accounting for other lifestyle and metabolic risk factors such as diabetes and high cholesterol.

> *Vegetarians were found to have a lower risk of developing gout, even when accounting for other lifestyle and metabolic risk factors.*

This research suggests that a plant-based diet could help prevent gout, and that these benefits are seen even in people who have high uric acid levels but not a formal diagnosis of gout. A vegetarian diet helps to reduce uric acid, while offering a wealth of nutrients crucial for overall health. Fruit and vegetable consumption usually leads to urine alkalization, which facilitates uric acid excretion in the urine.

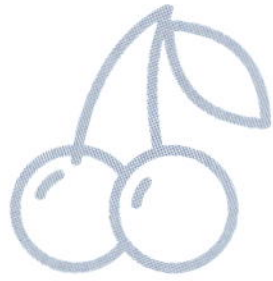

Cherries Are Special

In the 1950s, people began to report that eating cherries reduced their incidence of gout, triggering the interest of scientists. Recent research has shown that fresh cherries and their byproducts, such as cherry extract and cherry juice, can help lower the amount of uric acid in your bloodstream.

We still don't know why cherries have this beneficial effect. However, we do know that eating cherries can lower levels of C-reactive protein, a substance that plays an essential role in raising inflammation. Scientists think their gout-supportive benefits could also be due to the natural chemicals found in cherries. These include anthocyanins, a type of flavonoid with antioxidant and anti-inflammatory effects, that help people suffering with gout and prevent gout attacks.

One study involving more than 600 people suffering from gout who were followed over a period of one year revealed that those who ate cherries or consumed cherry extract experienced 35% fewer gout attacks compared to people not consuming the fruit. That's a significant decrease! The study further highlighted that this reduction was consistent across different demographics, gender, weight, the quantity of purines or alcohol intake and even in people using diuretics and drugs for gout.

In fact, when cherry consumption combined with the drug allopurinol, the risk of gout attacks dropped by an impressive 75%. However, because this study was based on observing people's habits and didn't control their behavior, we can only partially confirm that cherries were responsible for this benefit.

■ **Cherry Extract**

Since fresh cherries aren't available throughout the year, bottled tart cherry extract or juice is an accessible alternative. Pure tart cherry juice is the concentrated form of cherries, encapsulating all their beneficial compounds in a form that's easy to ingest.

One study of healthy people who were overweight and obese (and did not have a formal diagnosis of gout) found that those who drank a daily 8-ounce (240 mL) glass of tart cherry juice had a significant decline in their uric acid levels.

Additionally, a 2019 systematic review incorporating six studies found a recurring pattern: regular consumption of cherry products correlated with a decrease in both the incidence of gout attacks and their severity. Notably, tart cherry juice consumption was linked with decreased serum uric acid levels.

In September 2023, a randomized study looked at 282 men who did have a diagnosis of gout. These researchers found that using tart cherry juice decreased not only their uric acid levels, but also the frequency of their gout attacks and their markers of inflammation.

While many respected health organizations, such as the British Society for Rheumatology, European League Against Rheumatism, and National Institute for Clinical Excellence, recommend eating cherries to help with gout, some experts disagree. The Food and Drug Administration for instance, cautions people regarding claims that consuming cherry juice can treat gout.

My personal recommendation for patients with gout, in the absence of diabetes, is to consider eating 10 to 12 cherries daily when they are in season to potentially decrease the frequency of gout attacks. (See the *Gout Food Pyramid* on page 85).

While cherries might not be a magic bullet against gout, the prevailing evidence suggests they can be a valuable feature of a nutritious balanced diet, one building block of a comprehensive approach to managing gout, by decreasing uric acid levels and reducing gout flare-ups.

Fruits

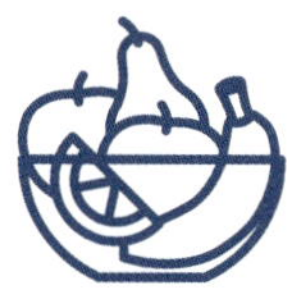

Eating more fruit is a good idea if you suffer from gout. In general, fruits provide a wide range of nutrients, including gut-supporting fiber, flavonoids and polyphenols.

Although there is some concern about eating fruit if you have gout, because it contains a lot of fructose and fructose metabolism can lead to urate, current research does not support this idea. The nutritional content of fruit is complex; fruits should not be seen only as a source of fructose.

One study of almost 30,000 males linked fruit consumption with a low prevalence of gout; less than 1% of 228 subjects were diagnosed with the condition. Although other variables weren't controlled for, this research suggests that the quantity of fruit you consume has an impact. People who averaged more than two pieces of fruit per day reduced their risk for gout by 50% compared with those who ate less than half a piece of fruit daily.

When you get to the *Gout Food Pyramid* (see page 85), you will see that fruits contain a wide variety of valuable nutrients with many different benefits and should be consumed daily.

CASE STUDY   **JAMES**

James, a 47-year-old slightly overweight African American male, was diagnosed with gout about three years ago. Initially he had attacks only in his big toe but, over time, other joints were affected. His attacks rotated among joints, traveling from his wrists and elbows to his knees and ankles. After diagnosis, James was started on allopurinol. He was consistent with his medication and his uric acid was close to the normal range thanks to his compliance.

However, he continued to experience gout attacks almost monthly. This took a toll on his mental well-being as he started to feel trapped by his body's unpredictable and painful reactions.

A friend recommended taking supplemental cherry extract. He called my office to ask for my opinion. I shared the results of a few studies and he decided to start taking cherry extract daily. Over the next six months, the frequency of his attacks declined, eventually ceasing entirely. For James, the combination of allopurinol and cherry extract seemed to be a winning formula.

Vegetables

Incorporating more vegetables into your diet can make a big difference if you have gout. Not only are vegetables low in purines, but they are also packed with nutrients and fiber.

A bounty of vegetables, especially leafy greens, bell peppers and broccoli, can be especially beneficial for those with gout. Leafy greens like spinach, kale, and Swiss chard are chock-full of vitamins A, C and K, and many B vitamins. Vegetables, like fruits and legumes, are loaded with fiber that will boost beneficial gut bacteria, improving uric acid metabolism in your body.

Eating a diet rich in vegetables and dairy can help with managing gout because these foods can make your urine more alkaline, which aids in flushing out uric acid.

Whole Grains

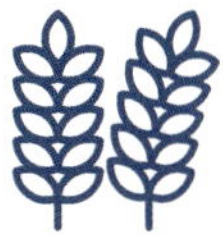

Whole grains are the seeds of certain plants. They differ from refined grains because they contain all three parts of the grain. When grains are refined, the bran and the germ are removed, leaving only the endosperm, the part that contains the fewest vitamins and minerals. Whole grains figure prominently in the Mediterranean dietary approach.

Among their benefits, whole grains offer a generous package of nutrients. They provide plant-based protein and healthy fats and are one of the best sources of dietary fiber. Although the nutrient content of individual grains varies, most whole grains contribute B vitamins (niacin, riboflavin, thiamine and folate), vitamin E, manganese and magnesium, plus a wide range of valuable phytonutrients. Many of these components help with managing gout.

Research shows that a diet rich in whole grains lowers the risk of gaining weight over time.

Three or more servings of whole grains every day has been shown to reduce your risk of developing obesity, type 2 diabetes and heart disease. As we know, gout is linked with all of these diseases. (You will see this recommendation for three servings a day in the *Gout Food Pyramid* on page 85.)

Whole Grains Provide Polyphenols

Fiber is just one of many, many nutrients provided by whole grains. They also provide vitamin E, folate and polyphenols. Among their benefits, polyphenols feed the "good guy" bacteria in your gut (see page 73). Polyphenols are also potent anti-inflammatories and antioxidants. Recent research suggests that that these anti-inflammatory and antioxidant effects can help with managing gout.

Refined Grains Lack Nutrients

Refined grains don't contribute the full range of vitamins, minerals, healthy fats, antioxidants and phytonutrients provided by whole grains. They also deliver far less fiber, most of which is concentrated in the missing bran layer. Moreover, when grains are refined, their natural balance shifts: the ratio of nutrients to calories is reduced. For instance, refined wheat (all-purpose white) flour provides only 59% of the folate provided by a comparable amount of whole wheat flour.

REFINED GRAINS AND CHRONIC DISEASE

Consumption of refined grains, including pasta, breakfast cereals, crackers and baked goods made with white flour, raises the risk of developing chronic illness. A 2021 study published in the *British Medical Journal* found that eating more than seven servings of refined grains daily increased your chances of having a stroke by 47%, and of developing heart disease by 33%. It also increased the likelihood of premature death by 27%.

Olive Oil

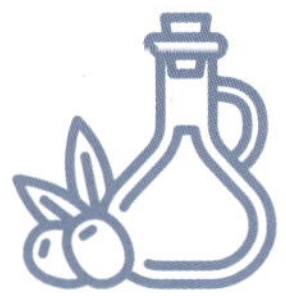

Olive oil, a staple of the Mediterranean diet since antiquity, has many well-documented health benefits, including potential to manage gout. Olive oil provides healthy fats such as omega-3s, which reduce inflammation—a critical aspect in managing gout attacks. Extra-virgin olive oil contains oleocanthal, which is a natural anti-inflammatory substance that appears to work in the body much like ibuprofen.

One Spanish study showed that olive oil supplementation and following a Mediterranean diet helped decrease uric acid blood levels, especially in patients with an increased risk of having a heart attack or stroke. The recommended dose was shown to be more than 4 tablespoons (60 mL) a day.

AIM FOR THE BEST

It pays to buy the best olive oil you can afford, because the least-processed oil provides the most health benefits. Look for cold-pressed extra-virgin olive oil, preferably unfiltered. Don't use your best olive oil for cooking.

Preferred Sources of Protein

Proteins play a pivotal role in our bodies, acting as essential building blocks for growth and repair. But when it comes to gout, not all proteins are created equal. When our bodies break down proteins, purines are produced. Some high-protein foods such as red meat and shellfish, which are high in purines, have been shown to increase uric acid, while others such as eggs and dairy don't have the same effect.

One study involving 2,000 individuals with gout found that participants who consumed high amounts of animal-based proteins had an elevated risk of developing gout. In contrast, those who ate more plant-based proteins, primarily from soy and legumes (beans, peas, lentils), had a decreased risk of the condition.

Dairy

Dairy products are a fantastic source of protein, among other valuable nutrients. Research suggests that consuming dairy products can help with managing gout. A U.S. survey of approximately 15,000 people showed that those who consumed milk at least once daily had a lower serum uric acid level than those who avoided milk. Similarly, those who consumed yogurt at least once every other day had a lower serum uric acid level than those who did not.

During a 12-year follow-up study, out of 14,000 men, about 700 developed gout. Men who consumed low-fat dairy products showed a 50% reduction in the risk of developing gout. These results were achieved by drinking two or more glasses of skim milk per day, or consuming low-fat yogurt, and were measured against men who drank less than one glass of milk per month.

I recommend to my patients that they consume one sugar-free, low-fat, plain yogurt daily. (See the *Gout Food Pyramid* at page 85.)

White Meat

Because meat is a source of high-quality protein, it can be a healthy addition to a plant-forward diet of nutritious whole foods. White meats such as chicken or turkey provide lean protein and have fewer purines than red meats, making them preferable.

Tofu: A Versatile Addition

Tofu is often used as a plant-based protein source. Studies have shown that consuming soy-based foods, including tofu, does not significantly increase the risk of gout or have clinically relevant effects on uric acid levels. Incorporating tofu and other soy-based foods into a gout-friendly diet helps reduce the intake of purine-rich foods associated with gout flare-ups.

Nuts and Seeds

In addition to being a good source of plant-based protein, nuts and seeds are nutritional powerhouses with many health benefits. Some, including walnuts, flaxseeds and chia seeds, are packed with omega-3 fatty acids, which are known for their potent anti-inflammatory effects. They are loaded with antioxidants such as vitamin E and minerals such as magnesium, zinc and selenium. It has been suggested that vitamin E and omega-3 fatty acids may also work together synergistically, boosting each other's anti-inflammatory and antioxidative effects.

A HANDFUL OF NUTS

A study published in 2018 showed that following the Mediterranean diet and eating a handful of nuts daily was potent in reducing cardiovascular risk and uric acid blood levels. About 44% of people could reduce their blood uric acid level using this approach. The study specifically recommended 30 g mixed nuts a day (15 g walnuts, 7.5 g almonds and 7.5 g hazelnuts).

Good and Bad Fats

Good fats usually refer to those associated with significant health benefits. These include mono- and polyunsaturated fats, including omega-3 fatty acids. These good fats are found in avocados, nuts, seeds, fish and olive oil, among other foods.

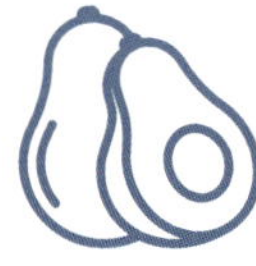

Some polyunsaturated fats (omega-6 fatty acids) are quite prevalent in the standard American diet. Research suggests that consumption of these fats, which are commonly found in vegetable and seed oils such as corn and sunflower oils, should be reduced, because we consume too many omega-6s relative to omega-3 fatty acids. Optimal proportions are no more than five-to-one ratio of omega-6 to omega-3. A low omega-3 to omega-6 ratio has been shown to trigger gout.

Saturated and trans fats are commonly called unhealthy fats. Saturated fats that are considered unhealthy, especially in large quantities, are found in animal products such as red and processed meats, and refined palm oil, an ingredient in many processed foods.

Although there have been serious efforts to reduce their presence in our food supply, trans fats (also called hydrogenated oils) are used in many processed foods, including some types of margarine and shortening, as well as fast foods. These fats are unhealthy because they have been shown to increase LDL (bad) cholesterol, while lowering HDL (good) cholesterol.

Fatty Fish

Eating fatty fish can be helpful for people with gout. Despite its higher purine content, some types of fish provide polyunsaturated fatty acids, specifically omega-3 fatty acids.

Research has proven eating foods high in omega-3s has many benefits for people with gout. Omega-3s inhibit the cyclooxygenase-2 (COX-2) enzyme. This is the same enzyme that, in NSAIDs (such as ibuprofen, diclofenac and naproxen), will inhibit and decrease in inflammation and pain. Because of this, foods with high omega-3 content will decrease inflammation.

A study of 724 people with gout found that those who ate fatty fish had a lower chance of getting recurrent gout attacks, while people taking omega-3s alone did not report this benefit.

Generally, seafood is high in purines. However, it differs in the amount of omega-3s it contains. Certain species of fish such as salmon and mackerel are naturally rich in omega-3 fatty acids, while shellfish are poor in omega-3 fatty acids.

Foods with a rich content of omega-3 fatty acids have anti-inflammatory benefits. This might help explain why there is an increased risk of gout and higher frequency of gout attacks when eating shellfish, but not when eating certain fatty fishes.

Omega-3 Rich		Omega-3 Poor	
Fish or Seafood Variety	EPA+DHA mg/ 4oz	Fish or Seafood Variety	EPA+DHA mg/ 4oz
Anchovies, herring	2300–2400	Catfish	100–250
Mackerel, Atlantic and Pacific (not king)	1350–2100	Clams	200–300
Oysters, Pacific	1550	Cod, Atlantic and Pacific	200
Salmon, Atlantic	1200–2400	Crab (blue, king, snow, queen)	200–550
Salmon (pink and sockeye)	700–900	Lobster	200
Sardines, Atlantic and Pacific	1100–1600	Mackerel (king)	450
Shark	1250	Scallops	200
Swordfish	1000	Shrimp	100
Trout (freshwater)	1000–1100	Squid	750
Tuna (albacore, canned)	1000	Tilapia	150
Tuna (bluefin, albacore)	1700	Tuna (canned)	150–300
		Tuna (yellowfin)	150–350

Adapted from American Heart Association, 2018

EAT FISH MORE OFTEN

If you are adhering to the Mediterranean dietary pattern, know that it suggests eating fish (not shellfish) that is abundant in omega-3 fatty acids (for example, salmon, trout, mackerel and sardines) at least three times a week. (See the *Gout Food Pyramid* on page 85.)

The Gout Food Pyramid

To make the information shared about food and gout in this chapter easier to visualize, I have created the Gout Food Pyramid, shown on the opposite page.

As you look from the bottom of the pyramid to the top, you will begin with the foods you should aim to consume on a daily basis, such as whole grains, leafy greens, fruits, plus a reminder to exercise and hydrate your body well.

Above these are "weekly" foods, such as legumes, eggs and fish, with notes on how many times a week you should consume them.

At the top of the pyramid are the foods and drinks you will want to have only sparingly, a few times per month, when you may want to indulge yourself with sweets or red meat or, more rarely, that glass of wine.

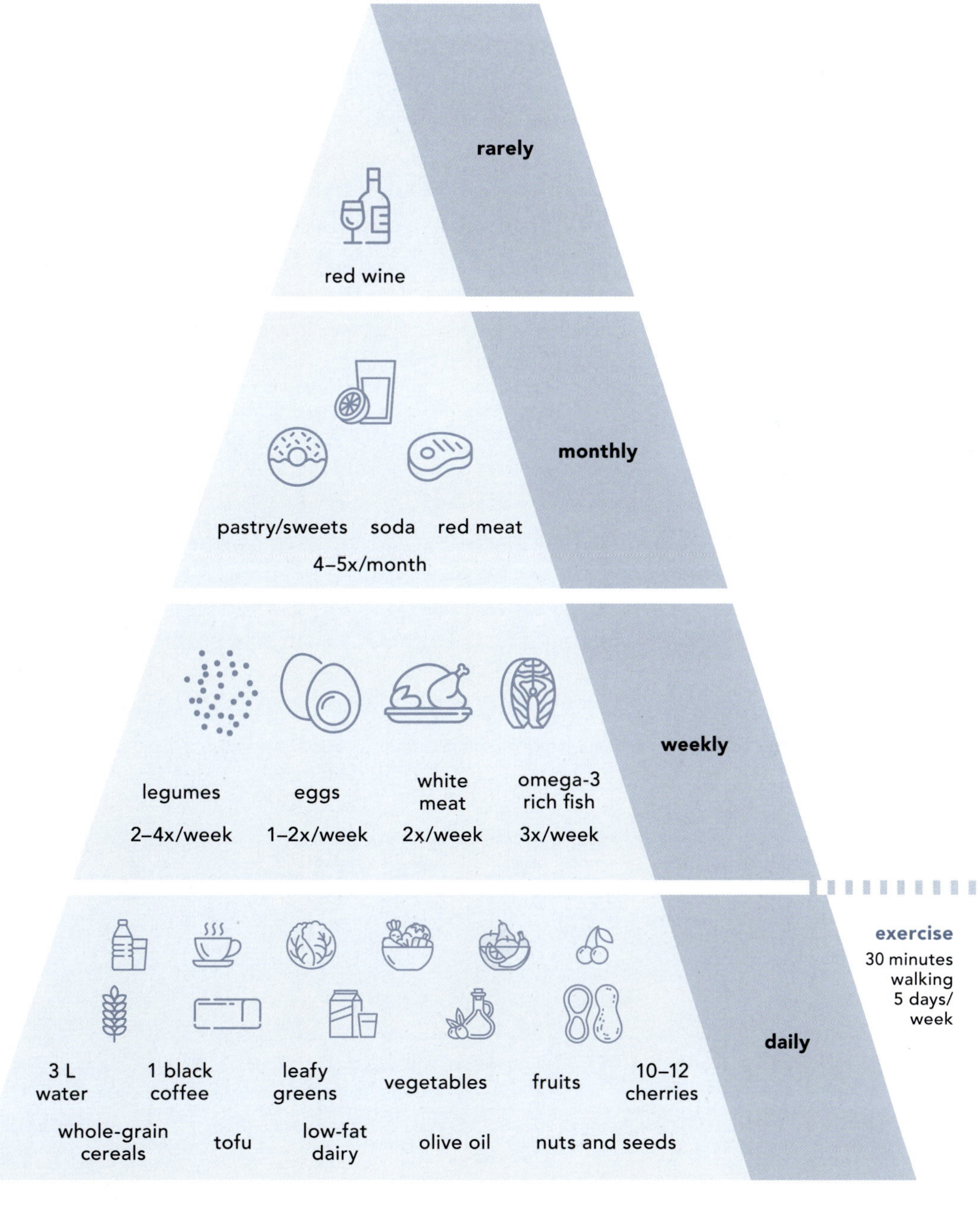

The Gout Food Pyramid, designed by Diana Girnita, adapted from the Mediterranean diet.
* People with a diagnosis of gout under control (meaning having a level of uric acid in the blood of less than 6.5 mL/dL and taking urate-lowering medication) should consume red wine rarely.

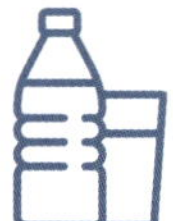

Staying Hydrated

Think of your body as a well-oiled machine in which uric acid is a byproduct of operating. When you're well hydrated, the machine functions smoothly and the uric acid you produce is flushed out in your urine. When you are dehydrated, you don't have enough fluid to rinse out the uric acid from your system. The result? Uric acid accumulates, crystallizes and settles in your joints, triggering a painful gout attack.

Drinking lots of water, especially after activities that spark dehydration by making you sweat, can help to keep your body running smoothly. In fact, a study found that gout sufferers who drank about eight cups of water in the 24 hours before a potential flare-up were less likely to have an attack. The study showed a 46% reduction in the risk of gout attacks.

You might be wondering if it's a good idea to substitute juice, soda or energy drinks for water. While these beverages might seem like a quick fix, they often contain added sugar or high-fructose corn syrup, which can boost uric acid production. They may also contain caffeine and/or salt, which can leave you more dehydrated than before.

DRINK WATER

An intense workout or spending too long in the sauna can make you dehydrated, which can trigger a gout attack. If you're planning a strenuous workout followed by a relaxing sauna, drink lots of water to stay hydrated.

Supplements

Throughout my years of practice, countless patients have asked about natural treatments for their health problems. The following information comes from my extensive literature search of the most commonly advertised supplements on the market: vitamin C, turmeric and omega-3s.

Vitamin C

Vitamin C is a multifaceted nutrient that supports many different processes in the body. It is well-known for its roles as an antioxidant, immune system enhancer and promoter of bone health. It also helps your body to metabolize protein.

Research shows that vitamin C can reduce uric acid levels through various mechanisms, including decreasing uric acid production and increasing its excretion in the kidneys.

Within the medical community there is an active debate regarding vitamin C supplementation for treating gout. There are studies that showed that, in people without a formal diagnosis with gout, the intake of vitamin C (around 500 mg/day) primarily from food sources will reduce uric acid levels, thus reducing the risk of developing the disease. Another study published in 2022 that included 14,000 males showed that vitamin C supplementation (of 500 mg/day) was associated with a 12% decrease in new gout diagnoses.

Within the medical community there is an active debate regarding vitamin C supplementation for treating gout.

This research suggests that vitamin C supplementation might be beneficial in decreasing uric acid in people with high blood levels of the substance.

However, studies in people with a formal diagnosis of gout did not show that vitamin C is beneficial. Thus, the American College of Rheumatology guidelines from 2020 do not support vitamin C supplementation in people with a diagnosis of gout.

Turmeric

Turmeric, a relative of ginger, is a vibrant, orange-colored root, commonly used in Asian cuisine such as curry dishes. Its therapeutic benefits are primarily attributed to its main active ingredient, curcumin.

Curcumin has traditionally been lauded for its robust anti-inflammatory and antioxidant activities, benefits which are now being confirmed by scientific research. Curcumin suppresses inflammation by blocking the same enzyme (COX-2) that conventional anti-inflammatory medications (NSAIDs) such as ibuprofen and naproxen use to reduce pain and inflammation.

A 2021 study of 39 participants exhibiting high uric acid levels, but without a formal gout diagnosis, showed a decline in uric acid levels with curcumin supplementation.

While we have many research studies that show the use of curcumin alleviates inflammation and pain in patients with rheumatoid arthritis and osteoarthritis, potentially reducing the need for conventional painkillers, the data for its efficacy in treating gout are still limited. The use of turmeric and curcumin supplementation might be beneficial for many reasons. However, if you supplement with curcumin supplementation solely to treat gout, be aware that it has not been scientifically proven to work.

Omega-3 Fatty Acid Supplements

As noted above, omega-3 fatty acids are essential because our body can't make them on its own. We need to get them from food or supplements. Since our diets aren't always perfect, taking a supplement seems like a viable and quick fix solution.

Omega-3 fatty acids have long been known as warriors against inflammation, so it's not surprising that people suffering from certain types of arthritis such as rheumatoid arthritis or osteoarthritis would find supplementing with omega-3s to be helpful. Most of these studies involved using fish oil supplements for at least 90 days, with a suggested dose of about 2 grams a day.

Omega-3s tame inflammatory arthritis. For instance, when people suffering from rheumatoid arthritis supplemented with omega-3 fatty acids (or fish oil) their pain and swelling was reduced, as was their need to use nonsteroidal anti-inflammatory medications.

Omega-3s tame inflammatory arthritis.

Omega-3 Supplements and Gout

If you do not like to eat fish, taking omega-3s supplements may appeal to you. Some studies suggest that if you have less omega-3s in your body, you might experience gout attacks more often. However, studies that compared the outcome based on the source of omega-3s (eating fish versus taking oral supplements) favored eating fish.

Another six-month study of 40 gout patients found that those taking a high dose of omega-3 fish oil (6.2 g) every day experienced fewer gout flare-ups. However, taking such a dose seems high. I'm concerned it could be potentially dangerous especially when combined with other medications.

Research has also shown promising connections between omega-3s and kidney health. One study from 2023 showed that people eating seafood with high content of omega-3s (fatty fish) seemed to have healthier kidneys and a lower risk of developing kidney disease. This is meaningful for gout sufferers, since the disease is frequently a consequence of kidney-related issues.

The research is inconsistent. While some studies that underscore the advantages of omega-3 supplementation, other studies do not support the practice. Nevertheless, in my view, if you don't like to eat fish and you have high cholesterol, high triglycerides or heart disease, it may make sense to use omega-3 supplements.

How Much Omega-3 Should I Take?

The FDA and NIH recommend a daily dose of 2 g of fish oil (omega-3 fatty acids) for most individuals. However, personal needs and reactions might differ. It's also important to be aware that fish oil can affect the absorption of specific medications, so check with your physician before supplementing.

CAUTION

Consult your health-care provider before adding any supplement to your regimen. One particular concern is that it may interact with your current medications.

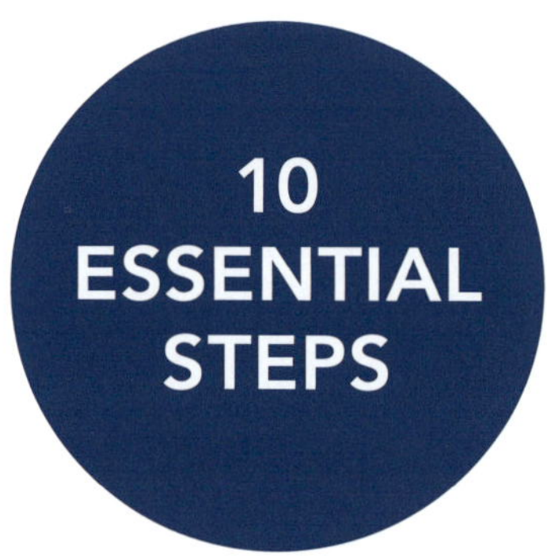

Living Your Best Life with Gout

Living with gout and managing its effects can often feel like navigating a labyrinth. Each turn offers new challenges and opportunities for understanding your condition and learning how to control it. This step-by-step guide will help you find your way more confidently.

■ STEP 1: Understand Your Condition

Gout is a unique form of arthritis. It is closely linked with your family history (genetics) and your current health. Gout frequently accompanies metabolic syndrome, a cluster of conditions that includes high blood pressure, high blood sugar and abdominal obesity.

■ STEP 2: Recognize the Signs

A gout attack is probably the most painful experience you will ever have. Gout attacks are most likely to originate overnight and first show up as redness and severe pain and swelling in your big toe. If left unchecked, these attacks will become increasingly frequent and expand their territory to include joints in different parts of your body. You ignore gout at your peril. Uncontrolled gout will leave its marks, translating to severe complications over time.

■ STEP 3: Get an Early Diagnosis

It's important to get a proper diagnosis as soon as possible. Without treatment your attacks will continue, worsening in severity and increasing in frequency. Early and consistent intervention prevents progression.

■ STEP 4: Understand the Role of Medication

Medication has an important role to play in managing gout. Being aware of the various approaches, both short term and long term, can help to keep gout under control. Treating co-existing conditions can also be helpful in managing gout. However, medication is not the only way to treat gout. Lifestyle interventions, from nutrition, to exercise and weight management, also play a crucial role in your successful battle against gout.

■ STEP 5: Stick with the Treatment Plan

Regular medical checkups are crucial if you have gout. Your uric acid levels need to be closely monitored and your physician needs to keep a close eye on whether the disease is progressing and treatment is effective.

■ STEP 6: Achieve a Healthy Weight

Being overweight is a major risk factor for gout as well as other chronic illnesses. Maintaining a healthy weight can help to prevent gout from developing and lessen its effect if it takes hold.

■ STEP 7: Know Your Triggers

Certain foods are high in purines, substances that can increase uric acid levels in your body. Identifying and avoiding these foods can help to prevent gout attacks. Other factors, including certain medications and becoming dehydrated, can also trigger gout.

■ STEP 8: Limit Alcohol Consumption

Understand how different kinds of alcohol influence gout and what that means for your lifestyle.

■ STEP 9: Discover Gout-Friendly Foods and Supplements

Numerous foods have been shown to help to prevent gout from developing and/or reduce its impact once it takes hold. Use the information in this book to explore foods and supplements that can be your allies in helping you to live better with gout.

■ STEP 10: Tweak Your Lifestyle

From weight loss and exercise to eating a more nutritious diet, scientific research suggests that lifestyle changes can reduce the risk and burden of gout. Use the recipes and meal plans in this book to help you maximize this potential.

CHAPTER 4

Food Journaling and Gout-Friendly Meal Plans

A FOOD JOURNAL can be instrumental in managing gout. Documenting what you eat can help you to identify and avoid the specific triggers that exacerbate your condition.

Over time, you can analyze this information to identify patterns and establish links between certain foods and the onset of gout symptoms.

Keeping a detailed record of what you eat is more valuable than you might think. Food reactions are highly personalized. Triggers can vary dramatically among individuals. Knowing what precipitates your flare-ups will go a long way toward helping you successfully manage gout.

Knowing what precipitates your flare-ups will go a long way toward helping you successfully manage gout.

Another benefit of food journaling is that it captures your behavior over time. This ongoing documentation can reveal unexpected patterns. It may, for instance, expose relationships between your emotions and what you eat.

Diligently documenting what you eat creates a detailed record of your customary choices. You may think your diet is healthy, but breaking it down by daily intake may disclose some not-so-good preferences or even bad habits.

For instance, we have long known that feeling stressed makes you hungry for junk food, which you may perceive as "comfort food." Ultraprocessed foods, such as packaged cakes and cookies, have been carefully calibrated to appeal to the pleasure centers in your brain. Enjoying some sweet treats may provide short-term emotional relief if you are feeling anxious, but it could also contribute to a gout attack.

When discussing a food diary with my patients, I suggest they make an initial commitment of a few weeks and then expand to a few months. The longer the time that you record, the better idea about your food habits you will have. You will have a higher chance to identify the triggers of your gout attacks.

How to Keep a Food Diary

An easy way to keep a food diary is to get a notebook and start recording what you eat during the day. It is best to record it immediately after you consume food, otherwise you might forget. You may also use the notes app in your smartphone. There are many applications that are compatible with your smartphone or tablet that can be very useful.

It is best to be as specific as possible and even write down the quantities of the food or drinks that you ingest.

FOOD DIARY TIP

A food diary must be accurate and consistent to serve its purpose effectively. A food diary isn't just for logging meals. Think of it as a mirror revealing your eating habits and choices, and the connections between your emotions and food.

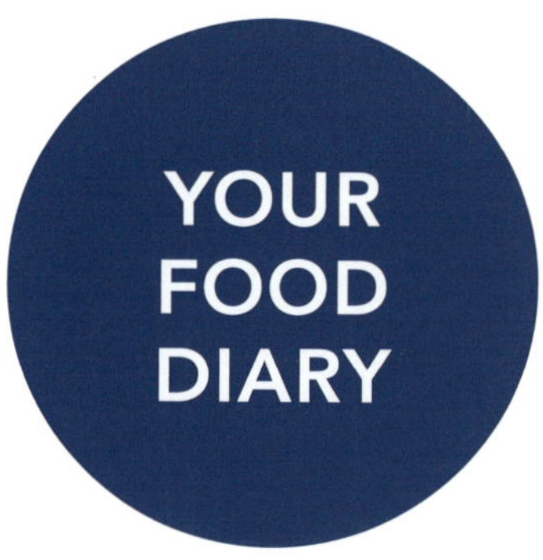

What Should You Include?

1 What you eat and drink

We have discussed in depth the triggers of gout attacks in *Chapter 2: Introducing Gout* and *Chapter 3: Living with Gout*. Be sure to record everything you eat and drink. You may start to notice patterns when you look back on what you have been eating and drinking.

2 How the food was prepared

For example, you may have fried potatoes, steamed vegetables or grilled fish. As we discussed in previous chapters, certain foods might become gout triggers when fried, as then they do contain more unhealthy fats. You may notice that eating fried chicken or fried potatoes triggers a gout attack, while eating baked chicken or potatoes does not.

❸ The quantity consumed, preferably using portions

Let's say you indulge in eating a cookie. That might not cause any harm, but eating five chocolate chip cookies at once can definitely increase the load of sugar and expose you to a gout attack. Similarly, eating a small piece of steak (4 oz/125 g) might not cause you any harm but having a big steak (14 oz/375 g) could set the stage for a gout attack.

❹ The timing of meals and snacks

Eating late at night, especially sugary snacks, will raise your blood sugar, increase the chances of weight gain and eventually increase your risk of developing gout or developing a gout attack.

❺ Where you are eating, with whom and if there are concurrent activities you are doing

For example, are you watching television? Eating at a party, or out with friends or while watching TV can be distracting and may lead to eating more food than you need. That is why paying attention to the environment is important, as it will influence your behavior.

❻ How you feel while you are eating

Did you feel anxious or depressed or did you feel happy? Many people tend to be influenced by their mood. Some people who are depressed tend to eat more, while others tend to eat less. For some, eating more or eating processed foods might be comforting. Some people, when they feel happy, tend to make better choices in the foods that they eat. They also are more likely to engage in exercising, which helps their overall health.

Some people benefit from organizing their meals and planning what will they have for breakfast, lunch and dinner. Staying on top of your schedule might look difficult in the beginning, but it will be very helpful in the long term.

Playing the Long Game: Set Goals

Once you've identified your gout triggers through your food diary, the next step is to set dietary goals that will help you to reduce the number of flare-ups you experience.

Trigger	Goal	Action
If you find that eating red or processed meat four times a week triggers a gout attack…	*Reduce red meat intake.*	Limit red meat consumption to no more than one serving per week for the next three months.
If you find that drinking sugary beverages (soda, juices, energy drinks) every day triggers a gout attack…	*Reduce sugary drink intake.*	Limit consumption of sugary drinks to no more than two times per week for the next three months.
If you find that organ meats (liver or kidneys) three times per week triggers a gout attack…	*Reduce the consumption of organ meats.*	Limit the intake of organ meats to once per month for the next six months.
If you find that drinking alcohol (especially beer) five times per week triggers a gout attack…	*Cut back on alcohol.*	Limit alcohol consumption to no more than twice a week for the next six months, and avoid beer.
If you find that eating seafood (shrimp, scallops, mussels) three times per week triggers a gout attack…	*Decrease seafood intake.*	Limit seafood intake to once a week for the next three months.

SET GOALS FOR SERVINGS

Type of Food	Goals for Servings
Vegetables	≥ 2 servings a day
Fresh fruits	≥ 2 to 3 servings a day
Legumes	≥ 3 servings a week
Fish	≥ 3 servings a week
White meat	Instead of red meat
Olive oil	≥ 4 tablespoons a day
Dairy, including milk, yogurt	1 cup a day
Nuts	≥ 3 servings a week
Commercially bakery goods, pastry and sweets	< 2 servings a week
Red meats	< 2 servings a week

Table designed based on information included in the PREDIMED Study 2018

Make a Meal Plan

A meal plan can be a valuable tool to help you improve your eating habits, achieve a specific health goal or manage a medical condition. Having a meal plan takes the guesswork out of what and what not to eat.

After following the meal plan for some time, eating well to manage gout will start to become second nature to you. By sticking to a gout-friendly meal plan, at least during the initial stage of managing it, you will develop healthy eating habits over time. This makes it easier to maintain a diet that supports gout management over the long run.

Sample Meal Plan

The meal plan that follows is structured to include daily recipes for a four-week period.

Because gout is a form of inflammatory arthritis caused by the accumulation of uric acid crystals in joints, the sample meal plan here includes recipes that are low in the dietary components of concern, including purines and fructose, both of which can aggravate gout and make its management difficult.

The meal plan also provides a pattern of eating that focuses on categories of foods that contain beneficial elements such as antioxidants, polyphenols and omega-3 fats that also help manage gout because they help to reduce inflammation. The recipes chosen include key foods that research has shown to benefit gout such as nuts, seeds, fish and legumes, plant-based entrées and, specifically, cherries, which have a unique role.

Rather than a focus on calories, protein, fat, fiber or portions, think of the meal plan as providing a pattern for your own gout-friendly eating habits. Including the recommended food categories in the book allows you the flexibility to create meals that suit you.

THE GOAL OF A MEAL PLAN

In the end, the goal of a meal plan is to provide consistency in your diet. Regular, balanced meals can help stabilize uric acid levels, reduce fructose intake and increase the intake of beneficial anti-inflammatory foods and nutrients helping to keep gout a manageable condition.

Gout-Friendly Meal Plan for Four Weeks

Meal Plan – Week 1

Meal	Sunday	Monday	Tuesday	
Breakfast	Cornmeal Crêpes with Avocado Filling	Spanish Potato Frittata	Pineapple-Coconut Overnight Oats	
Lunch	Chicken and Wild Rice Soup 1 slice of whole-grain bread	Health Wraps Ginger Pumpkin Soup	Egg Salad with Smoked Paprika	
Snack	Cherries	Plain yogurt with berries	Mixed nuts	
Dinner	Legume and Veggies Burger Salad* with Garlic Herb Vinaigrette	Chili-Glazed Salmon with Brussels Sprouts Simple Rice Pilaf	Chile Tofu and Green Beans Brown rice	

Meal Plan – Week 2

Meal	Sunday	Monday	Tuesday	
Breakfast	Fruit and Nut Breakfast Cookies	Garden Vegetable Frittata	Chicken Turnover Mixed berries	
Lunch	Roasted Eggplant and Feta Pizza Salad* with Lemon Cumin Dressing	Turkey Spinach Cobb Wrap Crunchy Fennel Salad	Gorgonzola Grinders Chickpea and Roasted Red Pepper Salad	
Snack	Orange	Mixed nuts	Cherries	
Dinner	Brine and Tender Lemon Roast Chicken Israeli Couscous with Mushrooms	Asian-Style Turkey Burgers All Greens Salad with Lemon Vinaigrette	Pork Tenderloin* with Charred Corn Salad Roasted Lemon Asparagus	

*Pork: Limit to 85 g per serving, about the size of a deck of cards

Wednesday	Thursday	Friday	Saturday
Crunchy Peach Parfait	Forbidden Black Rice with Coconut	Lox Scramble 1 slice of whole-grain toast	Apple Yogurt Chia Power Breakfast
Barley Chicken Salad	Classic Tuna Sandwich Three-Pea and Mint Salad	Veggie and Goat Cheese Wraps Tuscan White Bean and Tomato Salad	Turkey Spinach Cobb Wrap Southwest Slaw
Hummus with bell peppers	Cherries	Orange	Mixed nuts
Whole Wheat Pasta with Spring Vegetables and Edamame	Bok Choy, Tofu, and Shiitake Stir-Fry Brown rice	Roast Chicken Quarters with Lemon-Dill Spring Vegetables	Roasted Salmon and Root Vegetables with Horseradish

Wednesday	Thursday	Friday	Saturday
Ricotta Toast Grapefruit	Date Orange Muffin	Grape Oatmeal Cups Kiwi	Whole Wheat Cranberry-Orange Loaf
Chicken and Asparagus Wraps Roasted Carrot Soup with Pesto	Quinoa Bowl with Kale and Edamame	Fennel Salmon Salad Sandwich	Classic Tuna Sandwich Citrus Fennel Slaw
Fruit: pineapple, papaya or mango	Mixed berries	Hummus with veggies	Cheese and whole-grain crackers (feta, ricotta, no processed cheese)
Broiled Halibut and Pepper Skewers with Pesto Butter Toasts Honey Roasted Carrots	Chicken Mole Quinoa Pilaf Oven-Roasted Mixed Veggies	Lentil-Stuffed Eggplant Ginger and Orange Braised Carrots	Mushroom-Spinach Lasagna with Goat Cheese Green Salad with Garlic Herb Vinaigrette

Meal Plan – Week 3

Meal	Sunday	Monday	Tuesday	
Breakfast	Shakshuka with Chickpeas and Spinach	Cheddar 'n' Chive Scones	Cherry, Almond and Kale Smoothie	
Lunch	Crispy Baked Falafel Crunchy Fennel Salad	Veggie and Goat Cheese Wraps Roasted Carrot Soup with Pesto	Tofu Sandwiches with Tomatoes, Lettuce and Avocado	
Snack	Cherries	Plain yogurt	Cherries	
Dinner	Pasta with Chicken and Vegetable Sauce	Grilled Fish Skewers All Greens Salad with Lemon Vinaigrette	Green Pad See Ew	

Meal Plan – Week 4

Meal	Sunday	Monday	Tuesday	
Breakfast	Peach Crumbles with Greek Yogurt	Garden Vegetable Frittata	Big Batch Bran Muffins Banana	
Lunch	Grilled Fish Sandwich Southwest Slaw	Warm Italian Wraps Higher Morels Creamy Mushroom Soup	Egg Salad with Smoked Paprika Grilled Corn and Lima Bean Salad	
Snack	Fruit	Plain yogurt	Mixed nuts	
Dinner	Chicken Florentine with Wild Rice	Warm Kale, Tomato and Chickpea Salad Quinoa Pilaf	Fish and Spinach Tenga Rice	

Wednesday	Thursday	Friday	Saturday
Great Grains, Fruit and Nut Granola with Honey and Almond Butter	Green Tea Smoothie Bowel with Raspberries	Lox Scramble 1 piece of whole-grain toast	Maple Cinnamon Breakfast Quinoa
Fennel Salmon Salad Sandwich Higher Morels Creamy Mushroom Soup	Gorgonzola Grinders Chickpea and Roasted Red Pepper Salad	Turkey Spinach Cobb Wrap Roasted Carrot Soup with Pesto	Tofu and Bok Choy with Gingery Black Beans Rice
Mixed nuts	Fresh fruit	Mixed nuts	Hummus with bell peppers
Bok Choy, Tofu, and Shiitake Stir-Fry Brown rice	Whole Wheat Pasta with Spring Vegetables and Edamame	Chicken Florentine with Wild Rice Sautéed Red Chard with Lemon and Pine Nuts	Fettuccine with Fennel and Artichokes

Wednesday	Thursday	Friday	Saturday
Avocado Toast with Tomato Plain yogurt	Toasted Almond Muesli with Coconut and Chocolate	Apple Yogurt Chia Power Breakfast	Peanut Butter and Banana Oatmeal
Chicken Waldorf Sandwich Ginger Pumpkin Soup	Turkey Spinach Cobb Wrap	Classic Tuna Sandwich Crunchy Fennel Salad	Tomato, Fennel and Olive Pizza Warm Kale, Tomato, Chickpea Salad
Cherries	Mixed nuts	Cheese and whole-grain crackers	Fruit
Penne with Eggplant and Mushrooms	Southwestern Shepherd's Pie Steamed vegetables	Chicken and Vegetable Stew	Grilled Fish Skewers Buttery Garlic Mash Potatoes Stir-Fried Brussels Sprouts

Use This Book to Chart Your Course

Congratulations on completing this aspect of your journey, a giant step toward learning more about how you can effectively live with and manage gout.

In this book, I've tried to provided more than a superficial glance at the condition. I've worked hard to provide you with the most meaningful information about your condition and the steps you can take to keep it in check.

Gout isn't just a painful joint affliction that jolts you awake at night, or a short-term problem that disables you for days or a few weeks. It is a warning sign signaling that you have underlying metabolic problems that need to be addressed. With the insights from this book, you are armed with the knowledge and motivation to take control and change its course.

PART II

The
Recipes

CHAPTER 5

Breakfast

Great Grains, Fruit and Nut Granola with Honey and Almond Butter 106

Toasted Almond Muesli with Coconut and Chocolate 107

Grape Oatmeal Cups 108

Maple Cinnamon Breakfast Quinoa 109

Forbidden Black Rice with Coconut 110

Peanut Butter and Banana Oatmeal 111

Pineapple-Coconut Overnight Oats 112

Apple Yogurt Chia Power Breakfast 113

Crunchy Peach Parfaits 114

Peach Crumbles with Greek Yogurt 115

Cherry, Almond and Kale Smoothie 116

Spanish Potato Frittata 117

Garden Vegetable Frittata 118

Three-Cheese Potato Frittata 119

Shakshuka with Chickpeas and Spinach 120

Lox Scramble 121

Spinach-Mushroom Quiche 122

Mushroom Bread Cups 123

Cornmeal Crêpes with Avocado Filling 124

Ricotta Toast 125

Chicken Turnovers 126

Cheddar 'n' Chive Scones 127

Date Orange Muffins 128

Fruit and Nut Breakfast Cookies 129

Nut and Seed Breakfast Cookies 130

Whole Wheat Cranberry-Orange Loaf 131

Big Batch Bran Muffins 132

Pumpkin Loaf 133

Great Grains, Fruit and Nut Granola with Honey and Almond Butter

Joanne has been making this granola for years and always keeps a big jar on her kitchen island. Her teenage sons are elite athletes and can eat mountains of it.

Preheat oven to 325°F (160°C)

Rimmed baking sheet

TIPS

If you can't find barley flakes, use 6 cups (1.5 L) old-fashioned rolled oats.

To easily stir the oat-honey mixture, use clean hands lightly coated with oil. While it's baking, be sure to stir the oat mixture every 10 minutes to prevent the edges from burning. If you prefer larger chunks of granola, do not stir after it comes out of the oven for the final time.

To store, divide granola among airtight containers and store at room temperature for up to 1 month.

Joanne Rankin, Dietitian, British Columbia

½ cup	walnut halves	125 mL
½ cup	hazelnuts	125 mL
½ cup	almonds	125 mL
⅔ cup	almond butter or other natural nut butter	150 mL
½ cup	liquid honey	125 mL
2 tbsp	canola oil	30 mL
3 cups	old-fashioned rolled oats	750 mL
3 cups	barley flakes	750 mL
1 cup	wheat germ	250 mL
½ cup	ground flax seeds (flaxseed meal)	125 mL
1 tsp	vanilla extract	5 mL
½ cup	chopped dried apricots	125 mL
½ cup	raisins	125 mL
½ cup	chopped dates	125 mL

1 Spread walnuts, hazelnuts and almonds on baking sheet. Toast in preheated oven for about 15 minutes or until fragrant and lightly browned. Check often and stir during the final 5 minutes to avoid burning. Remove from oven, leaving oven on, and transfer nuts to a cutting board. Let cool completely, then coarsely chop.

2 In a medium, microwave-safe bowl, stir together almond butter, honey and oil. Microwave on High for about 1 minute or until bubbly. Set aside.

3 In a large bowl, stir together oats, barley flakes, wheat germ and flax seeds. Stir in hot honey mixture. Spread evenly on baking sheet.

4 Bake for 30 minutes. Every 10 minutes, remove from oven to stir, bringing grains from the outside to the center. Let cool completely on baking sheet on a wire rack.

5 Return to the bowl, sprinkle with vanilla and stir to combine. Stir in chopped nuts, apricots, raisins and dates.

Variation

You can vary the nuts and dried fruits, depending on preference and availability. This is also delicious with dried blueberries, cranberries and cherries.

Serving Idea

MAKE YOGURT PARFAITS: Place ¼ cup (60 mL) granola in a parfait or sundae glass. Layer with ½ cup (125 mL) chopped fresh fruit and ¾ cup (175 mL) yogurt. Sprinkle 2 tsp (10 mL) granola on top.

NUTRIENTS	CALORIES	FAT	CARBOHYDRATE	PROTEIN	FIBER
per serving	315	14.6 g	43 g	9 g	7 g

Toasted Almond Muesli with Coconut and Chocolate

Life is uncertain, so treat yourself to some chocolate for breakfast. Don't worry, despite the decadent taste, this muesli also packs a healthy dose of protein and whole-grain goodness. Enjoy it with sliced bananas and milk (dairy or non-dairy), or plain or vanilla-flavored yogurt (regular or Greek).

Preheat oven to 350°F (180°C)

18- by 13-inch (45 by 33 cm) rimmed sheet pan, lined with parchment paper

TIP

Store the cooled muesli in an airtight container at room temperature for up to 3 weeks or in the freezer for up to 3 months.

4 cups	large-flake (old-fashioned) rolled oats	1 L
1½ cups	sliced almonds	375 mL
1½ cups	unsweetened flaked coconut	375 mL
¾ tsp	salt	3 mL
3 tbsp	liquid honey	45 mL
3 tbsp	virgin coconut oil, warmed	45 mL
1 tsp	almond extract	5 mL
⅔ cup	miniature semisweet chocolate chips	150 mL

1. In a large bowl, whisk together oats, almonds, coconut and salt.

2. In a medium bowl, whisk together honey, coconut oil and almond extract until well blended.

3. Add the honey mixture to the oats mixture, stirring until well coated. Spread mixture in a single layer on prepared pan.

4. Bake in preheated oven for 15 to 20 minutes, stirring halfway through, until oats are light golden and almonds are toasted and fragrant. Let cool completely on pan.

5. Add the chocolate chips to the cooled muesli.

Nuts for Nutrition

Nuts are considered a meat alternative. A quarter cup (60 mL) is considered one serving. Nuts contain ample amounts of fat, so pay attention to portion size. For example, one handful of shelled roasted peanuts (about ½ cup/125 mL) provides just over 400 calories, with about three-quarters of the calories coming from fat.

NUTRIENTS	CALORIES	FAT	CARBOHYDRATE	PROTEIN	FIBER
per serving	310	19.3 g	29.7 g	6.9 g	6 g

Grape Oatmeal Cups

MAKES 6 SERVINGS

**SERVING SIZE:
2 OATMEAL CUPS**

Instead of a bowl of oatmeal, whip up your oats in handheld baked cups. This easy breakfast is quick to serve to kids with a glass of milk before school, and great to grab and go during a busy work week.

Preheat oven to 350°F (180°C)

12-cup muffin pan lined with paper cups and coated with nonstick cooking spray

TIP
For a creative twist, use ¾ cup (175 mL) seedless grapes, quartered, and ¾ cup (175 mL) strawberries, stems removed and thinly sliced.

3 cups	gluten-free large-flake (old-fashioned) rolled oats	750 mL
¼ cup	unsalted sunflower seeds	60 mL
1 tsp	baking powder	5 mL
1 tsp	ground cinnamon	5 mL
½ tsp	salt	2 mL
1½ cups	nonfat milk	375 mL
2	large eggs, beaten	2
¼ cup	pure maple syrup	60 mL
2 tbsp	unsalted butter, melted	30 mL
1 tsp	vanilla extract	5 mL
1½ cups	red or green seedless grapes, quartered	375 mL

1. In a medium bowl, mix together the oats, sunflower seeds, baking powder, cinnamon and salt.

2. In a large bowl, whisk together the milk, eggs, maple syrup, butter and vanilla extract.

3. Mix the dry ingredients into the wet ingredients until well combined. Fold in 1 cup (250 mL) of the grapes until evenly distributed.

4. Using a ¼ cup (60 mL), scoop the batter into each of the twelve muffin cups. Tap the muffin pan a few times on the countertop to release any air bubbles. Divide the remaining ½ cup (125 mL) grapes among the twelve cups.

5. Bake until the edges of the oat cups are slightly browned and a tester inserted into the center of one or two cups comes out clean, 45 to 50 minutes.

6. Remove the muffin pan from the oven and let cool for 15 minutes before transferring the oat cups to a wire rack to cool completely. Store at room temperature for up to 5 days.

NUTRIENTS	CALORIES	FAT	CARBOHYDRATE	PROTEIN	FIBER
per serving	329	11.2 g	48 g	11 g	5.1 g

Maple Cinnamon Breakfast Quinoa

MAKES 6 SERVINGS

Instant Pot

TIPS

When preparing foods that expand as they cook, such as quinoa, make sure to fill the pot no more than halfway full. Do not attempt to double or triple the recipe; otherwise, the exhaust valve may become clogged, resulting in excess pressure.

I used grapeseed oil in this recipe because it does not impart any additional flavors to the quinoa. However, you can use any other good/quality oil you have on hand.

Quinoa has a bitter coating that protects the grain. You may find pre-rinsed quinoa, but I still prefer to rinse it one more time to remove any bitter residue.

2 tsp	grapeseed oil	10 mL
1 cup	quinoa, rinsed	250 mL
¼ tsp	ground cinnamon	1 mL
Pinch	kosher salt	Pinch
2 cups	water	500 mL
2 tbsp	pure maple syrup	30 mL
1 tsp	vanilla extract	5 mL

1 Press Sauté on the Instant Pot; the indicator will read "Normal." When the display says "Hot," add oil to the pot and heat until shimmering. Add quinoa and cook, stirring, for 4 to 6 minutes or until golden brown. Press Cancel. Add cinnamon, salt, water, maple syrup and vanilla, stirring well.

2 Close and lock the lid and turn the steam release handle to Sealing. Press Manual; the indicator will read "High Pressure." Use the ⊖ button to decrease the time on the display to 1 minute.

3 When the timer beeps, press Cancel and let the pot stand, covered, for 10 minutes. After 10 minutes, turn the steam release handle to Venting and remove the lid.

4 Using a fork, fluff quinoa and transfer to serving bowls.

NUTRIENTS	CALORIES	FAT	CARBOHYDRATE	PROTEIN	FIBER
per serving	137	3.2 g	22.8 g	4 g	2.1 g

Forbidden Black Rice with Coconut

Black rice was once regarded as so superior in quality and nutritional value that it was reserved for Chinese royalty. Give yourself the royal treatment with this highly prized rice, crowned with toasted coconut and bananas.

Instant Pot

TIPS

When preparing foods that expand as they cook, such as rice, make sure to fill the pot no more than halfway full. Do not attempt to double or triple the recipe; otherwise, the vent pipe may become clogged, resulting in excess pressure.

Wash and rinse black rice two or three times. When washing, rub the rice grains together with your fingers to remove any excess starch and reduce clumping when cooked. Completely rinse the rice in a fine-mesh strainer under cold water.

Black rice is naturally chewier than white rice. If you want it to have a texture more like risotto, cover it with cold water and soak in the refrigerator for 4 hours or overnight. Rinse and drain thoroughly before adding to the pot.

1 cup	forbidden black rice, rinsed (see Tips)	250 mL
Pinch	kosher salt	Pinch
¾ cup	water	175 mL
⅔ cup	coconut milk, divided	150 mL
½ tsp	almond extract	2 mL
½ cup	unsweetened flaked coconut	125 mL
1	banana, sliced	1

1 In the inner pot, combine rice, salt, water, ½ cup (125 mL) coconut milk and almond extract, stirring well.

2 Place the pot inside the cooker housing, close and lock the lid and turn the steam release handle to Sealing. Press Manual; the indicator will read "High Pressure." Use the ➖ button to decrease the time on the display to 20 minutes.

3 Meanwhile, in a small skillet over high heat, toast coconut, stirring occasionally, for 3 minutes or until golden brown. Remove from heat and set aside.

4 When the timer beeps, press Cancel. Let stand, covered, until the float valve drops down. Turn the steam release handle to Venting and remove the lid.

5 Stir rice thoroughly. Divide rice among serving bowls and top with banana and toasted coconut. Drizzle with the remaining coconut milk.

NUTRIENTS	CALORIES	FAT	CARBOHYDRATE	PROTEIN	FIBER
per serving	686	30.4 g	96.2 g	9.9 g	9.2 g

Peanut Butter and Banana Oatmeal

MAKES 2 SERVINGS

This creamy oatmeal breakfast with its crowd-pleasing flavors of peanut butter and banana is a great way to start your day. Power up with this nourishing breakfast bowl, and you will feel like you can tackle anything.

Instant Pot

4-cup (1 L) heatproof bowl

Steam rack

TIP
You can use frozen sliced bananas in place of fresh, if desired.

⅔ cup	large-flake (old-fashioned) rolled oats	150 mL
½ cup	banana slices (about ½ banana)	125 mL
⅛ tsp	salt	0.5 mL
1⅓ cups	milk	325 mL
2 tbsp	peanut butter (approx.)	30 mL
1 tsp	packed brown sugar (optional)	5 mL

1 In the heatproof bowl, combine oats, banana slices, salt and milk.

2 Add 2 cups (500 mL) hot water to the inner pot and place the steam rack in the pot. Place a crisscross foil sling (see below) on the rack and place the bowl in the sling.

3 Close and lock the lid and turn the steam release handle to Sealing. Set your Instant Pot to pressure cook on High for 7 minutes.

4 When the cooking time is done, press Cancel and let stand, covered, until the float valve drops down, then remove the lid. The oatmeal should be creamy. (If more cooking time is needed, continue pressure cooking on High for 1 minute, then quickly release the pressure.)

5 Using the foil sling, remove bowl from the pot and immediately stir in peanut butter until well incorporated. Taste and add more peanut butter, if desired.

6 Divide oatmeal between serving bowls and sprinkle with brown sugar, if desired.

Crisscross Foil Sling

When you are steaming food inside a bowl or dish that fits very snugly in the pot and is deep enough that it would be difficult to use the handles of the steam rack to remove it from the pot, create a crisscross foil sling to help you lift the dish or bowl out.

It's easy to make a crisscross sling. Simply fold two 18-inch (45 cm) lengths of foil lengthwise into thirds, making two strips. Crisscross the center points of the strips on the steam rack, bringing the ends of the strips up the sides of the pot and over the rim. Place the bowl or dish on the crisscrossed strips on the rack and tuck the strip ends into the pot before closing and locking the lid. When the cooking time is done, grip the strip ends to lift out the bowl or dish. These foil strips can be reused several times, so store them with your Instant Pot for easy retrieval.

NUTRIENTS per serving	CALORIES	FAT	CARBOHYDRATE	PROTEIN	FIBER
	304	13.1 g	36.4 g	13 g	4.5 g

Pineapple-Coconut Overnight Oats

Overnight oats are a simple, no-cook way to ensure that you have breakfast ready to go all week long. The tropical flavors in this dish are perfect for summer, or for a little bit of sunshine any time of the year.

Five 16-oz (500 g) glass jars with lids

TIP
If you prefer, swap the same amount of pineapple for fresh or frozen mango.

2½ cups	gluten-free large-flake (old-fashioned) rolled oats	625 mL
3⅓ cups	nonfat milk	825 mL
5 tsp	sugar-free maple syrup	30 mL
5 tbsp	unsweetened shredded coconut	75 mL
1¼ cups	fresh or frozen and thawed pineapple chunks	310 mL
10 tbsp	sliced almonds	150 mL

1 In a large bowl, combine the oats, milk, maple syrup and coconut flakes.

2 TO STORE: Among five jars, divide the oats mixture. In each of five small sealable containers or zip-top plastic bags, add ¼ cup (60 mL) of the pineapple. In five additional small sealable containers or zip-top plastic bags, add 2 tbsp (30 mL) of the almonds. Cover or seal and refrigerate overnight and up to 5 days.

3 TO SERVE: Add the pineapple and almonds to the oatmeal and stir to combine. Enjoy cold or warm the oatmeal without the toppings in the microwave uncovered on High for 1½ to 2 minutes. Top with the pineapple and almonds after reheating.

Dairy Benefits

Dairy products are a fantastic source of protein, which helps your body grow and repair. Plus, they contain essential nutrients like calcium for strong bones and teeth. Yogurt, cheese or milk products provide a delicious way to fuel your body and keep you healthy and strong. Research has shown that incorporating milk, yogurt or cheese into your diet can decrease uric acid in your blood.

NUTRIENTS	CALORIES	FAT	CARBOHYDRATE	PROTEIN	FIBER
per serving	328.94	11.92 g	45.32 g	8 g	7.02 g

Apple Yogurt Chia Power Breakfast

MAKES 4 SERVINGS

The flavors of a warm apple pie meld together in this comforting, powered-up breakfast.

Instant Pot

TIP

When preparing oatmeal or any type of porridge using the Manual Pressure or Porridge functions, make sure to fill the pot no more than halfway full. Do not attempt to double or triple the recipe; otherwise, the exhaust valve may become clogged as the porridge froths up under pressure.

1 tbsp	butter	15 mL
1 cup	steel-cut oats	250 mL
1	large firm sweet apple (such as 1 Gala or Rome), peeled and diced	1
2 tbsp	packed light brown sugar	30 mL
1½ tsp	ground cinnamon	7 mL
¼ tsp	kosher salt	1 mL
3½ cups	water	875 mL
¼ cup	chia seeds	60 mL
¼ cup	plain Greek yogurt	60 mL
¼ cup	chopped walnuts	60 mL

1 Press Sauté on the Instant Pot; the indicator will read "Normal." When the display says "Hot," add butter to the pot and heat until melted. Add oats and cook, stirring, for 3 to 5 minutes or until fragrant. Press Cancel. Add apple, brown sugar, cinnamon, salt and water, stirring well.

2 Close and lock the lid and turn the steam release handle to Sealing. Press Manual; the indicator will read "High Pressure." Use the ⊖ button to decrease the time on the display to 3 minutes.

3 When the timer beeps, press Cancel. Let stand, covered, until the float valve drops down. Turn the steam release handle to Venting and remove the lid.

4 Stir oats. Stir in chia seeds. Cover and let stand for 5 minutes or until oats are desired consistency.

5 Divide oats among serving bowls, top each with a dollop of yogurt and sprinkle with walnuts.

Chia Seeds

Chia seeds offer much-needed fibers for smooth digestion (11 grams of fiber per ounce) and omega-3s to combat inflammation.

NUTRIENTS	CALORIES	FAT	CARBOHYDRATE	PROTEIN	FIBER
per serving	248	11.9 g	31.6 g	6.2 g	6.6 g

Crunchy Peach Parfaits

**MAKES 4 SERVINGS
(MAKES 2 CUPS/500 ML
GRANOLA)**

**SERVING SIZE: ¼ CUP
(60 ML) YOGURT, ¼ CUP
(60 ML) PEACHES WITH
JUICE, ¼ CUP (60 ML)
GRANOLA**

Parfaits are layers of yogurt, fruit and granola or nuts—a variety of flavors and textures in every bite. Fresh or canned peaches work beautifully in this recipe.

Preheat oven to 300°F (150°C)

Rimmed baking sheet lined with parchment paper

TIPS

If you prefer, swap the cashews for your favorite nut, like almonds, pistachios or walnuts.

Oats are naturally gluten-free, but some brands process their oats in a facility that also processes products with gluten. Check the label of your oats to make sure it was manufactured in a facility that is gluten-free.

HOMEMADE GRANOLA

¾ cup	gluten-free large-flake (old-fashioned) rolled oats	175 mL
¼ cup	raw or unsalted roasted cashews, coarsely chopped	60 mL
3 tbsp	unsalted sunflower seeds	45 mL
2 tbsp	unsweetened shredded coconut	30 mL
2 tbsp	sugar-free maple syrup	30 mL
1 tbsp	canola oil	15 mL
¼ tsp	vanilla extract	1 mL
¼ tsp	ground cinnamon	1 mL
⅛ tsp	kosher salt	0.5 mL
1	large egg white	1
2 tbsp	dried tart cherries	30 mL

PARFAITS

2½ cups	nonfat plain Greek yogurt	625 mL
2 cups	Homemade Granola	500 mL
2½ cups	no-sugar-added canned peaches, with juice	625 mL

1. **TO MAKE HOMEMADE GRANOLA:** In a medium bowl, mix together the oats, cashews, sunflower seeds, coconut, maple syrup, oil, vanilla, cinnamon and salt.

2. In a small bowl, whisk the egg white until frothy. Gently fold the egg white into the oats mixture, distributing it evenly.

3. Spread the granola in a single layer on the prepared baking sheet. Bake, using a spatula to turn sections of the granola over and breaking up larger pieces halfway through, until the granola is slightly browned and dried, 30 to 35 minutes.

4. Transfer the baking sheet to a cooling rack and let cool completely. Once cool, use a spatula to break up any larger pieces of the granola. Sprinkle in the tart cherries and gently toss to distribute.

5. **TO ASSEMBLE THE PARFAITS:** In each of four jars, add ¼ cup (60 mL) of the yogurt. Top with ¼ cup (60 mL) of the canned peaches with juice and about ¼ cup (60 mL) of the granola. Repeat the layers one more time, ending with the granola.

NUTRIENTS	CALORIES	FAT	CARBOHYDRATE	PROTEIN	FIBER
per serving	244	10.78 g	22.20 g	16.16 g	2.97 g

Peach Crumbles with Greek Yogurt

MAKES 4 SERVINGS

Try these buttery, pecan-stuffed peaches for a simple but impressive morning meal. A generous dollop of Greek yogurt adds creamy, protein-powered flair.

The nuts, spice, sweetener and fat in this recipe are all variable, so use what you have on hand or create your own favorite combinations. For example, for the nuts, try walnuts, almonds or pistachios. Use ground allspice, ginger or cardamom in place of the cinnamon. Try pure maple syrup, agave nectar or packed brown sugar for the sweetener, and consider olive oil or virgin coconut oil, melted, in place of the butter.

Preheat oven to 400°F (200°C)

18- by 13-inch (45 by 33 cm) rimmed sheet pan, lined with parchment paper or foil

TIP
Large firm-ripe nectarines can be used in place of the peaches.

4	large firm-ripe peaches	4
1 cup	large-flake (old-fashioned) or quick-cooking rolled oats	250 mL
⅓ cup	chopped pecans	75 mL
½ tsp	ground cinnamon	2 mL
⅛ tsp	salt	0.5 mL
5 tbsp	liquid honey, divided	75 mL
3 tbsp	unsalted butter, melted	45 mL
8 tbsp	plain or vanilla-flavored Greek yogurt	120 mL

1 Slice peaches in half vertically and remove pits. Arrange peaches, cut side up, on prepared pan, spacing evenly.

2 In a small bowl, combine oats, pecans, cinnamon and salt. Add 3 tbsp (45 mL) honey and butter, stirring until coated. Pack each peach hollow with oat mixture, dividing evenly.

3 Bake in preheated oven for 15 to 20 minutes or until peaches are softened and filling is golden brown. Let cool on pan on a wire rack for 5 minutes.

4 Top each peach half with 1 tbsp (15 mL) yogurt and drizzle with the remaining honey.

Dairy for Protein

Plain, unflavored yogurt is a great addition to your meal plan. Here are some examples of dairy products and their protein content per serving:

- **Greek yogurt:** 20 grams of protein per 1 cup (250 mL)
- **Cottage cheese:** 28 grams of protein per 1 cup (250 mL)
- **Milk:** 8 grams of protein per 1 cup (250 mL)
- **Cheddar cheese:** 7 grams of protein per 1 ounce (30 g)
- **Skim milk powder:** 1.5 grams of protein per 1 tablespoon (15 mL)

NUTRIENTS per serving	CALORIES	FAT	CARBOHYDRATE	PROTEIN	FIBER
	150	6.9 g	21.3 g	2.7 g	2.2 g

Cherry, Almond and Kale Smoothie

MAKES 2 SERVINGS.

SERVING SIZE:
1¼ CUPS (310 ML)

Kale is a green leafy
vegetable brimming
with vitamins and
minerals.

Blender

TIP
Remove any thick stems
from the kale before
using.

1½ cups	pitted frozen cherries	375 mL
1 cup	roughly chopped curly kale (see Tip)	250 mL
2	pitted dates	2
¾ cup	vanilla nonfat Greek yogurt	175 mL
¾ cup	unsweetened almond milk or nonfat milk	175 mL
2 tbsp	almond butter	30 mL

1 In a blender, combine the cherries, kale, dates, Greek yogurt, almond milk and almond butter; blend on high speed until smooth, about 1 minute.

2 Divide evenly between two glasses and serve immediately.

Cherries

These tasty fruits come in two main types: sweet cherries that you enjoy fresh during the summer and tart cherries that you can eat dried or squeezed into juice all year round, Cherry extract has been proven to reduce uric acid levels and decrease risk of gout attacks. For more about their nutritional value, see pages 76–77.

NUTRIENTS per serving	CALORIES	FAT	CARBOHYDRATE	PROTEIN	FIBER
	325	10 g	48 g	15 g	7 g

Spanish Potato Frittata

An adaptation of the Spanish potato omelet, this frittata is at home at breakfast, lunch or supper.

Preheat oven to 350°F (180°C)

2 tbsp	olive oil, divided	30 mL
1	small Spanish onion, chopped	1
2	cloves garlic, finely chopped	2
6	eggs	6
3 cups	diced cooked potatoes (about 3 medium)	750 mL
¾ tsp	salt	4 mL
¼ tsp	paprika	1 mL
¼ tsp	black pepper	1 mL

1. In a skillet, heat 1 tbsp (15 mL) oil over medium-high heat. Add onion and garlic. Cook, stirring occasionally, until softened and slightly golden, about 4 minutes.

2. In a large bowl, beat eggs. Add onion mixture, potatoes, salt, paprika and pepper.

3. Brush a 9-inch (23 cm) pie plate (preferably nonstick) with remaining 1 tbsp (15 mL) olive oil. Pour in egg mixture.

4. Bake in preheated 350°F (180°C) toaster oven for 30 minutes, or until eggs are set. Let stand for 5 minutes before cutting into wedges.

Serving Suggestion

If you wish, add ½ cup (125 mL) fresh or frozen and defrosted corn kernels to the egg mixture. Serve with chorizo sausage and sliced tomatoes. It is even good served cold.

NUTRIENTS	CALORIES	FAT	CARBOHYDRATE	PROTEIN	FIBER
per serving	217	11.2 g	19.5 g	9.8 g	2.5 g

Garden Vegetable Frittata

This makes a beautiful main course or side dish on a buffet, especially during spring and summer, when vegetables are at their peak of ripeness and flavor.

Preheat oven to 350°F (180°C)

11- by 7-inch (28 by 18 cm) glass baking dish, greased

TIP
Shocking vegetables in ice water stops the cooking process after blanching and sets the color, so you will have brightly colored vegetables even after baking.

1 lb	asparagus, trimmed and cut into 1-inch (2.5 cm) pieces	500 g
	Ice water	
1 tbsp	olive oil	15 mL
4 oz	mushrooms, sliced	125 g
1	clove garlic, minced	1
1	shallot, minced	1
1	small zucchini, cut in half lengthwise and thinly sliced	1
6	eggs	6
⅓ cup	milk	75 mL
1 tbsp	chopped chives	15 mL
1 tsp	salt	5 mL
½ tsp	freshly ground black pepper	2 mL
⅛ tsp	ground nutmeg	0.5 mL
2	tomatoes, thinly sliced	2
¼ cup	freshly grated Parmesan cheese	60 mL

1 In a large pot of boiling water, blanch asparagus for 1 to 2 minutes. Immediately plunge into ice water; let stand until chilled. Drain and place in prepared baking dish.

2 In a skillet, heat oil over medium heat. Sauté mushrooms for about 10 minutes or until tender. Add garlic and shallot; sauté for 2 minutes. Spread over asparagus. Arrange zucchini on top.

3 In a large bowl, whisk eggs until blended. Whisk in milk, chives, salt, pepper and nutmeg. Pour evenly over vegetable mixture. Arrange tomatoes on top. Sprinkle evenly with cheese.

4 Bake in preheated oven for 40 to 45 minutes or until set.

NUTRIENTS per serving	CALORIES 151	FAT 8.8 g	CARBOHYDRATE 8.5 g	PROTEIN 11 g	FIBER 2.7 g

Three-Cheese Potato Frittata

This hearty potato and cheese frittata supplies all of the energy you need for a weekend full of adventure (including reading about one while lounging in your favorite chair). Try it with sweet potatoes, too, or a combination of vegetables.

Preheat oven to 425°F (220°C)

18- by 13-inch (45 by 33 cm) rimmed sheet pan, lined with foil and sprayed with nonstick cooking spray

TIPS

For the best texture and flavor, choose regular or lower-fat ricotta cheese instead of nonfat.

Store cooled frittata squares in an airtight container in the refrigerator for up to 3 days or in the freezer for up to 3 months.

5 cups	diced peeled white or red round waxy potatoes	1.25 L
2 tbsp	olive oil	30 mL
¾ tsp	salt, divided	3 mL
¾ tsp	freshly ground black pepper, divided	3 mL
12	large eggs	12
1 tsp	baking powder	5 mL
1	container (16 oz/500 g) ricotta cheese	1
½ cup	milk	125 mL
⅓ cup	all-purpose flour	75 mL
8 oz	Gruyère or Swiss cheese, shredded	250 g
1 cup	grated Parmesan cheese	250 mL
½ cup	chopped fresh chives	125 mL

1. On prepared pan, toss potatoes with oil, ¼ tsp (1 mL) salt and ¼ tsp (1 mL) pepper. Spread in a single layer. Roast in preheated oven for 20 to 25 minutes or until potatoes are tender. Remove pan from oven and reduce heat to 350°F (180°C).

2. Meanwhile, in a large bowl, whisk together eggs, baking powder, and the remaining salt and pepper until blended. Whisk in ricotta and milk until blended and smooth. Stir in Gruyère, Parmesan and chives. Pour evenly over potatoes, smoothing top.

3. Bake for 30 to 35 minutes or until frittata is browned and puffed and a tester inserted near the center comes out clean. Let cool in pan on a wire rack for at least 20 minutes before cutting into squares. Serve warm or at room temperature.

NUTRIENTS	CALORIES	FAT	CARBOHYDRATE	PROTEIN	FIBER
per serving	395	23.7 g	22.4 g	23 g	1.8 g

Shakshuka with Chickpeas and Spinach

MAKES 5 SERVINGS

SERVING SIZE: 1¼ CUPS (310 ML) SHAKSHUKA WITH 1 EGG, ½ PITA

Shakshuka is a Mediterranean dish that cooks eggs in a tomato, pepper and onion sauce. This version adds more vegetables and legumes to make it even more nutritious.

TIP

If you prefer, swap the chickpeas for low-sodium white cannellini or red kidney beans. Both work beautifully in this recipe.

1 tbsp	olive oil	15 mL
1	large yellow onion, cut into ½-inch (1 cm) strips	1
1	red bell peppers, cut into 1-inch (2.5 cm) strips	1
1	clove garlic, minced	1
1	can (28 oz/796 mL) no-salt-added crushed tomatoes, with juice	1
1¾ cups	low-sodium canned chickpeas, drained and rinsed	425 mL
1 tbsp	chopped fresh cilantro or 1 tsp (5 mL) dried cilantro	30 mL
¼ tsp	salt	1 mL
¼ tsp	ground black pepper	1 mL
3 cups	baby spinach	750 mL
5	large eggs	5
2½	large (8-inch/20 cm) whole wheat pitas, halved (5 pieces)	2½

1   In a large sauté pan, heat the oil over medium heat. When the oil is shimmering, add the onion and bell peppers and sauté until softened, about 5 minutes. Add the garlic and cook until fragrant, about 1 minute.

2   Stir in the crushed tomatoes with juice, chickpeas, cilantro, salt, black pepper and Thai chile sauce. Increase the heat to medium-high and bring the mixture to a boil, then reduce the heat to medium-low. Add the spinach and stir to combine. Cover the pan and simmer, stirring occasionally, for about 10 minutes to let the flavors blend.

3   Using a wooden spoon, create a well in the tomato mixture along the outer edge of the pan. Break 1 egg into a small bowl or glass and gently pour into the well. Repeat with the remaining 4 eggs to form a circle along the outer edge of the pan. Reduce the heat to low, cover and cook until the eggs are set, about 6 minutes.

4   **TO STORE:** In each of five containers, add 1¼ cups (310 mL) of the shakshuka (including 1 egg). Wrap the pita halves individually in plastic wrap or aluminum foil and store on the side. Cover the containers and refrigerate for up to 4 days or freeze for up to 2 months.

5   **TO SERVE:** If frozen, thaw in the refrigerator overnight. To reheat the shakshuka with the egg, microwave uncovered on High for 60 to 90 seconds. Allow 2 minutes for the heat to distribute before removing the container from the microwave. Serve warm with a pita half.

NUTRIENTS per serving	CALORIES 327.68	FAT 10.18 g	CARBOHYDRATE 44.89 g	PROTEIN 17.59 g	FIBER 11.23 g

Lox Scramble

MAKES 2 SERVINGS

SERVING SIZE: ¾ CUP (175 ML)

Change up your morning scramble by adding bite-size pieces of lox or smoked salmon and green onions. It's not only easy with minimal prep but it's also delicious!

TIPS

There's no need to add salt to this recipe since the smoked salmon has plenty.

To make the dish lighter, swap an egg for 2 egg whites. You can do this with up to half the eggs in the recipe.

4	large eggs	4
2 oz	lox or cold-smoked salmon, chopped	60 g
1	green onion (whites and greens), chopped	1

PANTRY ITEMS

⅛ tsp	ground black pepper	0.5 mL
1½ tsp	olive oil	7 mL

1. In a medium bowl, whisk together the eggs and pepper.

2. Heat the oil in a large skillet over medium-low heat. When the oil is shimmering, pour the egg mixture into the center of the skillet. Cook the eggs, using a rubber spatula to push them gently from the edges into the center of the skillet, until they are almost set, 2 to 3 minutes. Stir in the salmon and green onions, cooking until eggs are cooked through, an additional 1 to 2 minutes. Serve immediately.

NUTRIENTS	CALORIES	FAT	CARBOHYDRATE	PROTEIN	FIBER
per serving	209	14.1 g	1.4 g	17.9 g	0.2 g

Spinach-Mushroom Quiche

MAKES 8 SERVINGS

This recipe is quick and easy, as it uses a prepared pie crust, which you can find in the refrigerator or freezer section of your supermarket.

Preheat oven to 425°F (220°C)

TIP
As the quiche bakes, you may need to cover the edges of the crust with foil to prevent excess browning.

1		9-inch (23 cm) unbaked pie shell	1
3		eggs	3
1 cup		milk	250 mL
½ tsp		salt	2 mL
½ tsp		freshly ground black pepper	2 mL
¼ tsp		ground nutmeg	1 mL
2 tbsp		butter	30 mL
2 cups		sliced mushrooms	500 mL
2 cups		shredded Swiss cheese	500 mL
1		package (10 oz/300 g) frozen chopped spinach, thawed and squeezed dry	1

1 Prick pie shell all over with a fork. Bake in preheated oven for 5 to 10 minutes or until lightly browned. Let cool slightly. Reduce oven temperature to 350°F (180°C).

2 In a medium bowl, whisk eggs until blended. Whisk in milk, salt, pepper and nutmeg.

3 In a skillet, melt butter over medium heat. Sauté mushrooms for about 5 minutes or until tender. Let cool slightly.

4 Add mushrooms, cheese and spinach to egg mixture and stir until combined. Pour into pie crust.

5 Bake in preheated oven for 1 hour or until a knife inserted in the center comes out clean.

NUTRIENTS	CALORIES	FAT	CARBOHYDRATE	PROTEIN	FIBER
per serving	316	21.2 g	18.8 g	13.3 g	1.8 g

Mushroom Bread Cups

Creamy mushrooms baked in bread cups make an attractive side dish for bacon and eggs, but these can also be served as a starter. The "cream" is actually cheese that melts during baking.

6	slices white or whole wheat sandwich bread, crusts removed	6
2 tbsp	olive oil, divided	30 mL
2 cups	sliced mushrooms (about 8 oz/250 g)	500 mL
1	clove garlic, finely chopped	1
3	green onions, chopped	3
¼ tsp	salt	1 mL
¼ tsp	black pepper	1 mL
⅔ cup	crumbled chèvre (goat cheese)	150 mL

1. Flatten bread slices with a rolling pin. Fit into six lightly greased muffin cups. Brush with 1 tbsp (15 mL) olive oil. Bake in preheated 350°F (180°C) toaster oven for 5 minutes. Remove from oven.

2. Meanwhile, in a large skillet, heat remaining 1 tbsp (15 mL) oil over medium-high heat. Add mushrooms and garlic. Cook, stirring occasionally, for 6 to 8 minutes, or until moisture has evaporated. Cool for 15 minutes. Stir in green onions, salt and pepper.

3. Place half of cheese in bottom of bread cups. Divide mushroom mixture evenly over cheese. Top with remaining cheese.

4. Return to oven and continue to bake for 20 minutes, or until edges of bread are golden and cheese has melted.

Make Ahead

Toast cups can be prepared up to 4 hours ahead and left at room temperature. Mushrooms can be cooked ahead and left at room temperature for an hour before assembling.

NUTRIENTS per serving	CALORIES 204	FAT 11.5 g	CARBOHYDRATE 16.7 g	PROTEIN 9 g	FIBER 1.4 g

Cornmeal Crêpes with Avocado Filling

MAKES 4 TO 6 CRÊPES

SERVING SIZE: 1 CRÊPE

Thicker than ordinary crêpes but thinner than pancakes, these cornmeal treats offer a unique taste and texture, resembling soft tacos.

6-inch (15 cm) crêpe pan or nonstick skillet

TIPS

Select an avocado that is firm to the touch yet yields with gentle pressure.

If the batter is too thick to spread, add another 1 tbsp (15 mL) milk.

If you find you cannot swirl the batter quickly enough for it to reach the edges of the pan, simply use more batter.

Laura Glenn, Dietetic Student, Quebec

CORNMEAL CRÊPES

½ cup	all-purpose flour	125 mL
⅓ cup	cornmeal	75 mL
1 tsp	baking powder	5 mL
1 tsp	granulated sugar	5 mL
¼ tsp	salt	1 mL
2	eggs	2
1 cup	low-fat plain yogurt	250 mL
3 tbsp	2% milk	45 mL
2 tbsp	melted non-hydrogenated margarine	30 mL
	Vegetable cooking spray	

AVOCADO FILLING

1	large ripe avocado	1
2 tsp	freshly squeezed lemon or lime juice	10 mL
2	ripe tomatoes, seeded and finely chopped	2
½ cup	chopped green onions	125 mL
1 tsp	chile and garlic sauce	5 mL
¼ tsp	salt	1 mL
¼ tsp	freshly ground black pepper	1 mL
¼ cup	low-fat sour cream (optional)	60 mL

1. **CRÊPES:** In a large bowl, combine flour, cornmeal, baking powder, sugar and salt.

2. In another large bowl, whisk together eggs, yogurt, milk and margarine. Make a well in the center of the flour mixture and gradually add the egg mixture, whisking until batter is blended and smooth. Cover and let rest at room temperature for 10 minutes.

3. Heat crêpe pan over medium heat. Spray lightly with cooking spray. Lift the pan and pour in about ⅓ cup (75 mL) batter. Swirl the pan so the batter reaches the edges. Return to heat and cook for about 1 minute or until crêpe is no longer shiny on top and is very light golden on the bottom. Flip and cook for 30 to 60 seconds or until starting to turn golden. Transfer to a plate, cover with foil and keep warm. Repeat with the remaining batter, spraying pan and adjusting heat between batches as needed.

4. **FILLING:** In a small bowl, mash avocado. Sprinkle with lemon juice. Gently stir in tomatoes, green onions, chile and garlic sauce, salt and pepper.

NUTRIENTS per serving	CALORIES 235	FAT 12.7 g	CARBOHYDRATE 24 g	PROTEIN 8 g	FIBER 4 g

5 Divide filling among crêpes. Fold bottom edge of crêpe over filling, then fold top edge over bottom edge. Transfer to a serving plate, seam side down. Serve with a dollop of sour cream, if desired.

Variation

Fill these crêpes with black beans, salsa and cheese in place of the avocado filling.

Avocados are one of the few fruits that contain a substantial amount of fat. But unlike coconut (the fruit of the tropical palm tree), which contains mostly saturated fat, avocados provide mainly monounsaturated fat.

Ricotta Toast

MAKES 2 SERVINGS

SERVING SIZE: 1 TOAST

You may already love jam on your morning toast, but take it up a notch by adding ricotta cheese. This soft, spreadable cheese has a creamy texture and adds protein to your meal, which helps keep you more satisfied.

TIPS

To lighten up the dish, choose part-skim ricotta cheese.

To increase the fiber, choose a whole wheat brioche or other whole wheat bread.

¼ cup	ricotta cheese	60 mL
2	slices brioche bread, toasted	2
2 tbsp	blueberry jam	30 mL

1 Spread 2 tbsp (30 mL) of the ricotta cheese on each slice of toast. Spoon 1 tbsp (15 mL) of the blueberry jam into the center of the ricotta cheese. Serve immediately.

NUTRIENTS	CALORIES	FAT	CARBOHYDRATE	PROTEIN	FIBER
per serving	207	4.8 g	35.1 g	5.6 g	1.4 g

Chicken Turnovers

Frozen prepared puff pastry is so easy to use. Only half a package is needed for this recipe, so keep the remaining pastry frozen or use any defrosted within two days. These turnovers are basically a chicken salad tucked into puff pastry, but they look as if you have really been cooking. You can also use cooked turkey or ham in these turnovers. For a vegetarian version, in place of chicken, use canned black beans that have been rinsed and well drained.

Toaster oven

1 cup	diced cooked chicken	250 mL
½ cup	chopped celery	125 mL
1	green onion, chopped	1
¼ cup	mayonnaise	60 mL
1 tbsp	mango chutney	15 mL
¼ tsp	curry powder	1 mL
¼ tsp	salt	1 mL
½	14-oz (397 g) package frozen puff pastry, defrosted but cold	½
1	egg	1
1 tbsp	milk	15 mL

1. In a bowl, combine chicken, celery, green onion, mayonnaise, chutney, curry powder and salt.

2. On a lightly floured surface, roll pastry into a 10/inch (25 cm) square. Cut into 4 squares. Place one-quarter of filling in center of each square.

3. In a small bowl or measuring cup, beat together egg and milk. Brush edges of pastry with egg mixture.

4. Fold each pastry in half diagonally to encase filling, pressing to seal tightly. Place turnovers on ungreased oven pan and brush with egg mixture.

5. Place pan on inverted bottom rack and bake in preheated 375°F (190°C) toaster oven for 25 to 28 minutes, or until pastry is puffed, golden and flaky.

Make Ahead

Turnovers can be assembled up to 6 hours earlier, covered well and refrigerated until baking time. Brush with glaze just before baking.

NUTRIENTS	CALORIES	FAT	CARBOHYDRATE	PROTEIN	FIBER
per serving	460	32.9 g	26.2 g	14.5 g	1.6 g

Cheddar 'n' Chive Scones

MAKES ABOUT 12 SCONES

Preheat oven to 400°F (200°C)

Baking sheet, lined with parchment paper

TIPS

It is important to use very cold butter when making scones so that it is easier to distribute the fat evenly throughout the mixture.

Add to the bread basket and serve with soup, beef stew, roast ham, chili or with a salad for lunch.

2 cups	all-purpose flour	500 mL
1 tbsp	baking powder	15 mL
¾ tsp	salt	3 mL
⅓ cup	cold butter, cut into cubes (see Tip)	75 mL
1½ cups	shredded sharp (old) Cheddar cheese	375 mL
2 tbsp	chopped fresh chives or green onions	30 mL
1¼ cups	milk	310 mL

1 In a large bowl, combine flour, baking powder and salt. With a pastry blender or 2 knives, cut in butter until mixture resembles coarse crumbs. Stir in cheese and chives.

2 Add milk all at once, stirring lightly with a fork until a soft dough forms. Using ⅓ cup (75 mL) measure, drop dough onto baking sheet. Bake in preheated oven until golden, 18 to 22 minutes. Serve warm.

NUTRIENTS	CALORIES	FAT	CARBOHYDRATE	PROTEIN	FIBER
per serving	192	10.5	18 g	6.3 g	0.6 g

Date Orange Muffins

Serve these delicious lactose-free muffins for a light but nutritious start to the day. For a more wholesome muffin, substitute ½ cup (125 mL) whole wheat flour for ½ cup (125 mL) all-purpose flour.

1⅓ cups	all-purpose flour	325 mL
⅓ cup	packed brown sugar	75 mL
1 tsp	baking powder	5 mL
½ tsp	baking soda	2 mL
¼ tsp	salt	1 mL
½ cup	chopped pitted dates	125 mL
1	egg	1
1 tbsp	grated orange zest	15 mL
¾ cup	orange juice	175 mL
¼ cup	vegetable oil	50 mL
½ tsp	vanilla	2 mL

1 In a large bowl, combine flour, brown sugar, baking powder, baking soda, salt and dates.

2 In a separate bowl, beat egg. Beat in orange zest, orange juice, oil and vanilla. Add to dry ingredients and stir just to combine.

3 Spoon batter into six lightly greased muffin cups. Bake in preheated 375°F (190°C) toaster oven for 22 minutes, or until muffin tops are firm to the touch and golden. Turn pan halfway through baking time. Cool muffins in pan for 5 minutes before turning out onto a rack.

NUTRIENTS per serving	CALORIES 287	FAT 10.3 g	CARBOHYDRATE 45.3 g	PROTEIN 4.5 g	FIBER 1.9 g

Fruit and Nut Breakfast Cookies

MAKES 9 SERVINGS

SERVING SIZE: 1 COOKIE

You can enjoy diabetes-friendly cookies for breakfast! The trick is using whole grains, nuts and fruit in the batter so you have a medley of nutritious ingredients.

Preheat oven to 350°F (180°C)

2 baking sheets lined with parchment paper and coated with cooking spray

TIP
Rinse your hands in cool water before rolling the dough. The dough will be easier to roll and won't stick as much to your hands.

¾ cup	unbleached all-purpose flour	175 mL
¾ cup	100% whole wheat flour	175 mL
½ cup	large-flake (old-fashioned) rolled oats	125 mL
1 tsp	ground cinnamon	5 mL
1 tsp	baking soda	5 mL
¼ tsp	ground nutmeg	1 mL
¼ tsp	salt	1 mL
1	medium ripe banana, mashed	1
¼ cup	stevia brown sugar blend (such as Truvia or Splenda)	60 mL
¼ cup	canola oil	60 mL
1 tbsp	sugar-free maple syrup	30 mL
2	large eggs, beaten	2
1 tsp	vanilla extract	5 mL
¼ cup	shelled unsalted pistachios, coarsely chopped	60 mL
3 tbsp	raw walnuts, coarsely chopped	45 mL
¼ cup	dried tart cherries	60 mL
3 tbsp	dried apricots, chopped	45 mL

1. In a medium bowl, mix together the all-purpose flour, whole wheat flour, oats, cinnamon, baking soda, nutmeg and salt.

2. In a large bowl, whisk together the mashed banana, brown sugar blend, oil, maple syrup, eggs, and vanilla until the mixture is smooth and creamy.

3. Gently fold the dry ingredients into the wet ingredients and stir until just combined. Fold in the pistachios, walnuts, cherries and apricots, making sure to evenly distribute them throughout the batter.

4. Using clean hands, roll 3 tbsp (45 mL) of dough into a ball and place on a prepared baking sheet. Repeat with the remaining dough, leaving about 2 inches (5 cm) between cookies. Gently press down on the top of each cookie to flatten slightly.

5. Bake until the cookies are soft and golden brown and a tester inserted into the center of one or two cookies comes out clean, 15 to 18 minutes. Transfer the cookies to a wire rack and let cool for 5 minutes.

6. **TO STORE:** Place cookies in individual zip-top plastic bags and store them on the counter for up to week. Extra cookies can be stored in individual zip-top plastic bags in the freezer for up to 2 months.

7. **TO SERVE:** If frozen, thaw on the counter overnight. Serve at room temperature or warm. To reheat, place the cookie on a baking sheet in an oven preheated to 350°F (180°C) for about 5 minutes or until warmed through.

NUTRIENTS	CALORIES	FAT	CARBOHYDRATE	PROTEIN	FIBER
per serving	201.07	9.84 g	24.44 g	5.19 g	2.67 g

Nut and Seed Breakfast Cookies

MAKES 15 SERVINGS

SERVING SIZE 1 COOKIE

These breakfast cookies are brimming with immune-boosting ingredients: almonds, walnuts and sunflower seeds. Meal prep these cookies on Sunday and enjoy them throughout your busy work week. Pair with a glass of milk, yogurt or fresh fruit.

Preheat oven to 350°F (180°C)

2 baking sheets lined with parchment paper

1½ cups	unbleached all-purpose flour	375 mL
1 cup	large-flake (old-fashioned) rolled oats	250 mL
1 tsp	ground cinnamon	5 mL
1 tsp	baking soda	5 mL
½ tsp	salt	2 mL
1 cup	almond butter	250 mL
½ cup	unsweetened applesauce	125 mL
6 tbsp	pure maple syrup	90 mL
2	eggs, beaten	2
1 tsp	vanilla extract	5 mL
¼ cup	raw walnuts, coarsely chopped	60 mL
¼ cup	raw almonds, coarsely chopped	60 mL
¼ cup	unsalted sunflower seeds	60 mL
½ cup	raisins	125 mL

1. In a medium bowl, using a wooden spoon, mix together the all-purpose flour, oats, cinnamon, baking soda and salt.

2. In a large bowl, whisk together the almond butter, applesauce and maple syrup until well combined. Add the eggs and vanilla extract and whisk until smooth.

3. Gently fold the dry ingredients into the wet ingredients and stir until just combined. Fold in the walnuts, almonds, sunflower seeds and raisins, evenly distributing throughout the dough.

4. Scoop out ¼ cup (60 mL) of the dough and, using clean hands, roll into a ball. Place onto a prepared baking sheet and gently press down on the top to flatten slightly. Repeat with the rest of the batter, leaving about 1 inch (2.5 cm) between the cookies.

5. Bake for 18 minutes, until the cookies are golden brown but soft and a tester inserted into the center of two cookies comes out clean. Transfer the cookies to a wire rack and let cool for about 10 minutes.

6. Serve warm or, once the cookies have completely cooled, store, covered, at room temperature for up to 5 days. Cookies can also be placed in a sealable bag and stored in the freezer for up to 2 months.

NUTRIENTS per serving	CALORIES 258	FAT 14 g	CARBOHYDRATE 27.9 g	PROTEIN 7.8 g	FIBER 3.6 g

Whole Wheat Cranberry-Orange Loaf

SERVING SIZE 1 SLICE

Enjoy a delicious slice of this fruit-filled loaf. Cranberries are an excellent source of the antioxidants vitamins C and E and can be a delicious part of your immune-boosting diet.

9- by 5-inch (23 by 12.5 cm) loaf pan coated with nonstick cooking spray

	Juice of 1 navel orange and five 1-inch (2.5 cm) slices of orange peel	
1½ cups	dried cranberries	375 mL
1 cup	boiling water	250 mL
1 cup	unbleached all-purpose flour	250 mL
1 cup	100% whole wheat flour	250 mL
1½ tsp	baking powder	7 mL
½ tsp	baking soda	2 mL
½ tsp	salt	2 mL
½ cup	canola oil	125 mL
½ cup	low-fat (1%) milk	125 mL
⅓ cup	pure maple syrup	75 mL
¼ cup	light brown sugar	60 mL
2	large eggs, beaten	2
1 tsp	vanilla extract	5 mL

1. Add the orange peel and cranberries to a medium bowl and cover with the boiling water. Set aside and let soak for 1 hour.

2. Preheat the oven to 350°F (180°C).

3. In a medium bowl, sift together the all-purpose flour, whole wheat flour, baking powder, baking soda and salt.

4. In a separate medium bowl, whisk together the canola oil, milk, maple syrup and brown sugar. Whisk in the orange juice, eggs and vanilla.

5. Drain the cranberries and discard the orange peel.

6. Add the dry mixture to the wet mixture and stir until just combined. Gently fold in the cranberries until evenly distributed in the batter.

7. Pour the batter into the prepared loaf pan and use a spatula to even out the top. Bake until a tester inserted into the loaf comes out clean, 50 to 55 minutes. Remove from the oven and let cool for 10 minutes. Turn out onto a wire rack to cool completely.

8. Cut the loaf into eight equal slices. Serve immediately or store, covered, for up to 5 days. The loaf can also be stored in the freezer for up to 2 months.

Whole Wheat

Whole wheat flour offers 6 grams of fiber per cooked 1-cup (250 mL) serving. Adding fiber to your diet can benefit your gut microbiome, digestive health, weight management, blood sugar regulation and heart health. Feeling fuller for longer helps control appetite, aiding in weight loss or healthy weight maintenance, reducing obesity-related risks.

NUTRIENTS	CALORIES	FAT	CARBOHYDRATE	PROTEIN	FIBER
per serving	41	15.8 g	64.9 g	5.4 g	2.4 g

Big Batch Bran Muffins

The batter is prepared ahead and is ready to be scooped and baked as needed.

Muffin pan, greased or lined with paper muffin cups

TIPS

Measure oil first then honey and molasses. The sticky stuff will slip easily out of the measuring cup.

In all cake and muffin baking have your ingredients at room temperature before starting to mix for easy blending.

Wheat bran is the outer layer of the wheat kernel that is high in carbohydrates, calcium and fiber. Wheat germ is the highly nutritious core of the wheat kernel. We add bran and wheat germ to some of our breads, muffins, cookies and loaves for hearty nutty flavor and added health benefit.

6½ cups	natural bran (see Tips)	1.625 L
4 cups	whole wheat flour	1 L
7 tsp	baking soda	35 mL
1½ tsp	salt	7 mL
8	eggs	8
⅔ cup	packed brown sugar	150 mL
3 cups	buttermilk	750 mL
1⅓ cups	sunflower oil	325 mL
1½ cups	liquid honey	375 mL
1½ cups	light (fancy) molasses	375 mL

1 In a bowl, combine bran, flour, baking soda and salt. Set aside.

2 In a large bowl, whisk together eggs, brown sugar, buttermilk, sunflower oil, honey and molasses until smoothly blended. Add flour mixture. Mix well. Cover and refrigerate overnight or for up to 6 weeks.

3 Preheat oven to 400°F (200°C).

4 Spoon batter into prepared muffin cups, filling almost full.

5 Bake in preheated oven until top springs back when lightly touched, 20 to 25 minutes. Let cool for 10 minutes in pan on a wire rack, then remove from pan and let cool.

Variations

Add raisins, chopped dates or apricots to the mixture either when mixing or when ready to bake.

NUTRIENTS	CALORIES	FAT	CARBOHYDRATE	PROTEIN	FIBER
per serving	218	8.4 g	36. 6 g	4.8 g	2.3 g

Pumpkin Loaf

MAKES 1 LOAF

A sprinkling of toasted pumpkin seeds on top adds a pleasing crunch to this spicy moist loaf.

Preheat oven to 350°F (180°C)

9- by 5-inch (23 by 12.5 cm) loaf pan, greased and lined with parchment paper

TIP

Be sure to buy pumpkin purée not pumpkin pie filling. The pie filling has sugar and spices added to it.

1½ cups	all-purpose flour	375 mL
⅔ cup	granulated sugar	150 mL
1 tsp	baking powder	5 mL
1 tsp	baking soda	5 mL
1 tsp	ground cinnamon	5 mL
½ tsp	ground nutmeg	2 mL
½ tsp	ground cloves	2 mL
¼ tsp	salt	1 mL
2	eggs	2
1 cup	canned pumpkin purée (not pie filling) (see Tip)	250 mL
⅓ cup	sunflower oil	75 mL
½ cup	raisins	125 mL
2 tbsp	green pumpkin seeds	30 mL

1. In a bowl, combine flour, sugar, baking powder, baking soda, cinnamon, nutmeg, cloves and salt. Set aside.

2. In a large bowl, with a wooden spoon, beat together eggs, pumpkin and oil until smooth. Gradually add flour mixture, beating until blended. Stir in raisins. Spread batter evenly in prepared pan. Sprinkle pumpkin seeds over top.

3. Bake in preheated oven until tester inserted in center comes out clean, 55 to 60 minutes. Let cool for 15 minutes in pan on a wire rack, then remove from pan and let cool completely on rack.

NUTRIENTS	CALORIES	FAT	CARBOHYDRATE	PROTEIN	FIBER
per serving	259	9.3 g	41.3 g	4.2 g	3.3 g

CHAPTER 6

Lunch

Barley Chicken Salad — 136

Chicken Waldorf Sandwich — 137

Chicken and Asparagus Wraps — 138

Turkey Spinach Cobb Wraps — 139

Lamb Burgers with Cucumber-Mango Raita — 140

Cucumber-Mango Raita — 141

Asian-Style Turkey Burgers — 142

Classic Tuna Sandwich — 143

Grilled Fish Skewers — 144

Fennel Salmon Salad Sandwiches — 145

Quinoa Bowls with Kale and Edamame — 146

Sesame-Miso Garlic Dressing — 147

Egg Salad with Smoked Paprika — 148

How to Build and Bake a Pizza — 149

Roasted Eggplant and Feta Pizza — 150

Tomato, Fennel and Olive Pizza — 151

Tofu Sandwiches with Tomatoes, Lettuce and Avocado — 152

Baked Marinated Tofu — 153

Health Wraps — 154

Gorgonzola Grinders — 155

Veggie and Goat Cheese Wraps — 156

Crispy Baked Falafel — 157

Warm Italian Wraps — 158

Warm Kale, Tomato and Chickpea Salad — 159

Barley Chicken Salad

6 cups	water	1.5 L
	Salt to taste	
1 cup	pearl barley	250 mL
2 lbs	boneless skinless chicken breasts	1 kg
3	stalks celery, diced	3
1 cup	chopped walnuts	250 mL
1 cup	mayonnaise	250 mL
2 tbsp	tarragon vinegar	30 mL
2 tsp	dried tarragon	10 mL
1 tsp	brown mustard	5 mL
	Freshly ground black pepper to taste	

In a large pot, bring water and ½ tsp (2 mL) salt to a boil.

Add barley, reduce heat, cover and simmer for 20 minutes.

Add chicken, cover and simmer for 20 minutes, until chicken is no longer pink inside and barley is tender.

Drain, cut chicken into bite-size pieces and place in a serving bowl with barley, celery and walnuts.

Whisk together mayonnaise, vinegar, tarragon, mustard, pepper and additional salt; pour over salad and toss to coat.

Whole Grains

Whole grains can be part of salads, soups, or enjoyed as a side dish. Remember to drink plenty of water when increasing fiber intake to ensure smooth digestion. Fiber is a nutrient with great value in combating gout. Barley offers 6 grams of fiber per cooked 1-cup (250 mL) serving.

NUTRIENTS per serving	CALORIES	FAT	CARBOHYDRATE	PROTEIN	FIBER
	585	38.3 g	25.6 g	35.1 g	6 g

Chicken Waldorf Sandwich

This recipe is a twist on Waldorf salad. It's perfect to serve during the fall at the peak of apple and pecan season.

TIPS

I used Gala or Braeburn apples in this recipe but any sweet-tart apple will do. There's no need to peel them—the skin adds color and nutrition.

When purchasing lemons, look for ones that are plump, firm and heavy for their size.

3 tbsp	mayonnaise	45 mL
3 tbsp	low-fat apple-flavored or vanilla yogurt	45 mL
1 tbsp	freshly squeezed lemon juice	15 mL
2½ cups	chopped cooked chicken	625 mL
½ cup	chopped apples (see Tips)	125 mL
½ cup	diced celery	125 mL
½ cup	chopped pecans, toasted	125 mL
⅓ cup	dried cranberries or cherries	75 mL
8	slices whole wheat bread (½-inch/1 cm thick slices)	8
4	lettuce leaves	4

1 In a large bowl, stir together mayonnaise, yogurt and lemon juice. Add chicken, apples, celery, pecans and cranberries. Mix well. Cover and refrigerate for at least 30 minutes or for up to 2 days to allow flavors to blend and mixture to chill slightly.

2 Place bread slices on a work surface. Arrange lettuce over 4 of bread slices. Spread chicken salad equally over lettuce and cover with remaining bread.

NUTRIENTS per serving	CALORIES 533	FAT 26 g	CARBOHYDRATE 44.2 g	PROTEIN 32.3 g	FIBER 6.5 g

Chicken and Asparagus Wraps

MAKES 4 SERVINGS

This chicken and asparagus combination works great in a wrap sandwich. Spread with a Classic Aïoli and sprinkle with Parmesan cheese.

Preheat oven to 450°F (230°C)

Large rimmed baking sheet, greased

TIP

To warm tortillas, place on a plate, layered with paper towels, alternating paper towels and tortillas, covering top layer with a towel. Microwave on High for 10 to 20 seconds or until warm.

½ cup	freshly squeezed lemon juice (about 3 lemons)	125 mL
6 tbsp	olive oil, divided	90 mL
2	cloves garlic, minced	2
1 tsp	sea salt, divided	5 mL
½ tsp	freshly ground black pepper, divided	2 mL
1½ lbs	boneless skinless chicken cutlets or chicken tenders, cut into thin strips	750 g
1 lb	asparagus, trimmed and cut into 1-inch (2.5 cm) pieces	500 g
4	8-inch (20 cm) flour tortillas, warmed (see Tip)	4
	Classic Aïoli (page 211)	
½ cup	freshly grated Parmesan cheese	125 mL

TOPPINGS, OPTIONAL

Diced tomatoes
Arugula leaves

1 In a shallow dish, combine lemon juice, 2 tbsp (30 mL) of the olive oil, garlic, ¼ tsp (1 mL) each of the salt and pepper. Add chicken and coat well. Let stand at room temperature for 15 minutes or cover and refrigerate for up to 8 hours.

2 In a saucepan of boiling water, blanch asparagus for 2 minutes. Drain well. Arrange in a single layer on prepared baking sheet and sprinkle with remaining salt and pepper. Drizzle with 2 tbsp (30 mL) of olive oil. Bake in preheated oven for 6 to 8 minutes or until asparagus is tender. Set aside.

3 Meanwhile, in a large skillet, heat remaining oil over medium-high heat. Sauté chicken for 5 minutes or until no longer pink inside. Spread 1 tbsp (15 mL) Classic Aïoli equally along center of each tortilla. Arrange chicken, asparagus, Parmesan and desired toppings on top. Fold both edges over filling. Roll up and serve immediately.

Variation

Feel free to substitute thinly sliced turkey for the chicken in this sandwich.

NUTRIENTS	CALORIES	FAT	CARBOHYDRATE	PROTEIN	FIBER
per serving	614.3	31.4 g	34.2 g	49 g	13.8 g

Turkey Spinach Cobb Wraps

MAKES 4 SERVINGS

4	10-inch (25 cm) flour tortillas	4
2 cups	baby spinach leaves	500 mL
8 oz	thinly sliced deli turkey	250 g
8	bacon slices, cooked	8
2	tomatoes, thinly sliced	2
2	avocados, thinly sliced	2
1 cup	shredded Cheddar cheese	250 mL
2	hard-boiled eggs, thinly sliced	2
1 cup	ranch dressing	250 mL
1/8 tsp	salt	0.5 mL
1/8 tsp	freshly ground black pepper	0.5 mL

1 Place tortillas on a work surface. Arrange spinach, turkey, bacon, tomatoes, avocados, Cheddar cheese and eggs equally in center of each tortilla. Top each with ranch dressing and sprinkle with salt and pepper. Fold both edges over filling. Roll up and serve immediately.

NUTRIENTS per serving	CALORIES	FAT	CARBOHYDRATE	PROTEIN	FIBER
	972	66.5 g	56.6 g	40.2 g	24.9 g

Lamb Burgers
with Cucumber-Mango Raita

MAKES 4 SERVINGS

Lamb burgers are
great when you want
a "different" burger.
It is wonderful
topped with the
Cucumber-Mango
Raita.

**Preheat greased
barbecue grill to
medium-high**

**Instant-read
thermometer**

1½ lbs	lean ground lamb	750 g
1	clove garlic, minced	1
2 tbsp	finely chopped onion	30 mL
½ tsp	ground cumin	2 mL
½ tsp	paprika	2 mL
½ tsp	salt	2 mL
¼ tsp	freshly ground black pepper	1 mL
4	hamburger buns, split and toasted	4
4	Bibb lettuce leaves	4
	Cucumber-Mango Raita	

1 In a large bowl, combine lamb, garlic, onion, cumin, paprika,
   salt and pepper. Shape into 4 equal patties, about ¾ inch
   (2 cm) thick.

2 Place burgers on preheated grill, close lid and grill, turning
   once, for 4 to 6 minutes per side or until an instant-read
   thermometer registers 160°F (71°C). Serve on buns with lettuce
   and Cucumber-Mango Raita.

NUTRIENTS	CALORIES	FAT	CARBOHYDRATE	PROTEIN	FIBER
per serving	611	41.6 g	23.9 g	33 g	1.4 g

Cucumber-Mango Raita

**MAKES 1½ CUPS
(375 ML)**

**SERVING SIZE: 2 TBSP
(30 ML)**

TIP
When substituting fresh mint for dried, use three times as much fresh for the dried.

2	medium cucumbers, peeled, seeded and grated	2
1	medium mango, peeled and chopped	1
2 tbsp	freshly chopped mint	30 mL
2 tbsp	freshly chopped cilantro	30 mL
2 cups	plain Greek yogurt	500 mL
½ tsp	kosher salt	2 mL

1. In a large bowl, combine cucumber, mango, mint and cilantro. Stir in yogurt and salt and mix well. Use immediately or cover and refrigerate for up to 2 days.

Beware the Big Burger

Lamb burgers are good for a change, but should be consumed in moderation, less than once a week. This burger also works well with ground turkey or chicken. Beware: if you don't make your own burgers, but eat in a restaurant, portions may be big enough to precipitate a flare-up.

NUTRIENTS	CALORIES	FAT	CARBOHYDRATE	PROTEIN	FIBER
per serving	603	9.6 g	107.3 g	32.5 g	8.8 g

Asian-Style Turkey Burgers

MAKES 4 SERVINGS

These Asian burgers are wonderful served with a side of slaw with red and green cabbage and shredded carrots topped with sesame seeds.

Preheat greased barbecue grill to medium-high, if using

Instant-read thermometer

TIP
When you're trying to determine how much fresh ginger you will need, usually a 2-inch (5 cm) piece of ginger yields 2 tbsp (30 mL) minced.

1 lb	lean ground turkey	500 g
2	cloves garlic, minced	2
2 tbsp	finely chopped onion	30 mL
2 tbsp	finely chopped green bell pepper	30 mL
1 tsp	reduced-sodium soy sauce	5 mL
2 tsp	grated fresh gingerroot (see Tip)	10 mL
½ tsp	salt	2 mL
¼ tsp	freshly ground black pepper	1 mL
4	whole-grain hamburger buns, split and toasted	4

TOPPINGS, OPTIONAL
Lettuce
Tomato slices

1 In a large bowl, combine turkey, garlic, onion, bell pepper, soy sauce, ginger, salt and pepper. Shape into 4 equal patties, about ¾ inch (2 cm) thick.

2 Place patties on preheated grill, close lid and grill, turning once, for 6 to 8 minutes per side or until an instant-read thermometer registers 160°F (71°C).

3 Place buns on a work surface. Top with burgers, desired toppings and remaining buns.

Opt for White Meats
The Mediterranean diet often includes turkey and chicken breast as lean protein sources. These meats can be prepared in various ways, such as grilling, baking or sautéing. Choose white meats more often than red; white meats have less purine content, which is important because high purine levels can increase uric acid levels in the body, triggering gout attacks.

NUTRIENTS per serving	CALORIES	FAT	CARBOHYDRATE	PROTEIN	FIBER
	298	10.4 g	23.6 g	27 g	1.1 g

Classic Tuna Sandwich

MAKES 4 SERVINGS

TIP
Be sure to always drain
the liquid from the
canned tuna.

2	cans (each 6 oz/170 g) tuna, drained (see Tip)	2	
¼ cup	finely chopped celery	60 mL	
⅓ cup	Homemade Mayonnaise (page 210) or store-bought	75 mL	
¼ tsp	salt	1 mL	
¼ tsp	freshly ground black pepper	1 mL	
8	slices whole wheat or white bread (½-inch/1 cm thick slices)	8	
4	lettuce leaves	4	
4	small tomatoes, thinly sliced	4	

1 In a large bowl, combine tuna, celery, mayonnaise, salt and pepper. Cover and chill in the refrigerator for at least 30 minutes or for up to 1 day for flavors to blend.

2 Place bread slices on a work surface. Arrange lettuce, tuna and tomatoes over half of bread and cover with remaining bread slice.

Variations

Classic Tuna with a Twist: Add 1 tbsp (15 mL) pickle relish and 1 tsp (5 mL) grated lemon zest in Step 1. Proceed as directed.

Greek-Style Tuna: Omit celery. Add ¼ cup (60 mL) finely chopped red bell pepper, ¼ cup (60 mL) finely chopped green bell pepper, 2 tsp (10 mL) freshly squeezed lemon juice and ¼ cup (60 mL) chopped black olives in Step 1. Proceed as directed.

NUTRIENTS	CALORIES	FAT	CARBOHYDRATE	PROTEIN	FIBER
per serving	422	18.8 g	33.2 g	29.7 g	5.8 g

Grilled Fish Skewers

Fish recipes are limited in the land-locked northern states. Traditionally, local river fish would be used for this recipe, but any firm-fleshed fish will be suitable.

Bamboo skewers, soaked in water for 30 minutes

2 lbs	skinless firm fish fillets, such as catfish, snapper, redfish, halibut or cod	1 kg

MARINADE

1 cup	plain nonfat yogurt	250 mL
3 tbsp	chickpea flour (besan)	45 mL
2 tsp	minced garlic	10 mL
2 tsp	coriander powder	10 mL
1½ tsp	salt or to taste	7 mL
1 tsp	cumin powder	5 mL
1 tsp	turmeric	5 mL
1 tsp	cayenne pepper	5 mL
¾ tsp	carom seeds (ajwain)	4 mL
½ tsp	garam masala	2 mL
3 tbsp	freshly squeezed lime or lemon juice	45 mL
1 tbsp	oil	15 mL
	Additional oil for broiler pan or grill	
	Lemon wedges	
	Mint sprig	

1 Rinse fish and pat dry thoroughly. Cut into 1½-inch (4 cm) pieces.

2 MARINADE: In a large nonreactive bowl, whisk together yogurt, chickpea flour, garlic, coriander, salt, cumin, turmeric, cayenne, carom seeds and garam masala. Add lime juice and oil. Add fish and stir to coat with mixture. Set aside at room temperature for 15 minutes or refrigerate for up to 2 hours.

3 Thread 2 to 3 pieces on each skewer. Thread another skewer parallel to first, through pieces, so fish does not rotate on skewers. Discard remaining marinade.

4 Preheat broiler. Line broiler pan with foil and brush liberally with oil. Arrange skewers on pan and broil, turning once, 3 to 4 minutes. Alternatively, cook on a well-oiled preheated grill, turning once, 3 to 4 minutes. Garnish with lemon wedges and mint sprig.

NUTRIENTS	CALORIES	FAT	CARBOHYDRATE	PROTEIN	FIBER
per serving	141	2.9 g	3.7 g	24 g	0.6 g

Fennel Salmon Salad Sandwiches

3 tbsp	mayonnaise	45 mL
2 tbsp	freshly squeezed lemon juice	30 mL
1 tbsp	sour cream	15 mL
8	slices black bread	8
1 tbsp	chopped fennel leaf	15 mL
½ cup	finely diced fennel bulb	125 mL
2	cans (each 6 oz/170 g) salmon, drained	2
4	leaves Romaine lettuce	4

Combine mayonnaise, lemon juice and sour cream; spread 1 tsp (5 mL) of this sauce on each slice of bread.

In a large bowl, toss fennel leaf, diced fennel and salmon; combine with the remaining mayonnaise mixture.

Build 4 sandwiches using the salmon salad and 1 lettuce leaf per sandwich.

NUTRIENTS	CALORIES	FAT	CARBOHYDRATE	PROTEIN	FIBER
per serving	364	14.9 g	29.7 g	28.3 g	4.5 g

Quinoa Bowls with Kale and Edamame

MAKES 4 SERVINGS

Build a bowl and you are good to go for lunch. Packed in a tub, the pickled onion will soften and mellow by lunchtime. If making ahead, slice the avocado at the last minute so it will stay nice and green.

TIPS

If you prefer a hot lunch, you can reheat the quinoa before building the bowls.

Quick-pickled red onion gets better with time, so if you have an hour to let it sit and mellow, do so.

1 cup	slivered red onion	250 mL
2 tbsp	granulated sugar	30 mL
2 tbsp	apple cider vinegar	30 mL
½ cup	Sesame-Miso Garlic Dressing (page 147)	125 mL
1 tbsp	Sriracha	15 mL
3 cups	cooked quinoa	750 mL)
1	avocado, sliced	1
4 oz	baby kale, chopped	125 g
2 cups	frozen shelled edamame, thawed	500 mL
1 cup	drained roasted red peppers, slivered	250 mL
1 cup	pea sprouts (optional)	250 mL

1 Place onion in a medium bowl. Add sugar and vinegar, tossing to coat. Let stand at room temperature, stirring occasionally, for at least 10 minutes or up to 1 hour.

2 In a medium bowl or cup, stir together sesame-miso dressing and Sriracha.

3 Divide quinoa among four wide pasta bowls. Arrange pickled onion, avocado, kale, edamame, red peppers and pea sprouts (if using) on top, dividing evenly. Drizzle with dressing.

Variation

Use another flavorful sprout, such as daikon or broccoli, in place of the pea sprouts.

To Pack for Lunch

Build each bowl in a 3-cup (750 mL) food storage container, omitting the avocado and dressing. Divide dressing among 4 small airtight containers. Refrigerate for up to 1 day. In the morning, pit the avocado, cut it into quarters and sprinkle each with a few drops of apple cider vinegar; wrap each quarter tightly with plastic wrap. Refrigerate until serving. Pack an avocado quarter and a container of dressing along with each bowl. Slice and scoop avocado into the bowl and drizzle with dressing just before serving.

NUTRIENTS per serving	CALORIES 483	FAT 21 g	CARBOHYDRATE 58.6 g	PROTEIN 20.3 g	FIBER 14.2 g

Sesame-Miso Garlic Dressing

MAKES ABOUT 2½ CUPS (625 ML)

SERVING SIZE: 2 TBSP (30 ML)

This dressing does double duty as a sauce for just about anything, from stir-fries and grain bowls to wraps and noodles. The tahini, made from sesame seeds, adds protein and calcium, so drizzle freely and enjoy!

Blender (see Tip)

TIPS

In a pinch, you can make this dressing without a blender. Just mince the garlic and ginger and whisk in the remaining ingredients until smooth.

Try this with other kinds of miso. The darker a miso is, the more intense the flavor will be.

Leave out the garlic if you're worried about having garlic breath.

4	cloves garlic, chopped	4
2 tbsp	sliced gingerroot	30 mL
2 tbsp	packed brown sugar	30 mL
1 tsp	hot pepper flakes	5 mL
¾ cup	water	175 mL
¾ cup	tahini	175 mL
¼ cup	unseasoned rice vinegar	60 mL
2 tbsp	tamari	30 mL
2 tbsp	toasted (dark) sesame oil	30 mL
¼ cup	white miso	60 mL

1 In blender, combine garlic, ginger, brown sugar, hot pepper flakes, water, tahini, vinegar, tamari, sesame oil and miso; blend until smooth, scraping down the sides of the container as needed.

2 Transfer dressing to a jar or other airtight container and store in the refrigerator for up to 1 week.

NUTRIENTS	CALORIES	FAT	CARBOHYDRATE	PROTEIN	FIBER
per serving	80	6.3 g	4.5 g	2.2 g	0.7 g

Egg Salad with Smoked Paprika

MAKES 4 SERVINGS

The hint of smoked flavor works wonderfully in this egg salad recipe.

8	large eggs	8
	Cold water	
	Ice cubes	
2 tbsp	Homemade Mayonnaise (page 210) or store-bought	30 mL
2 tbsp	minced chives	30 mL
½ tsp	smoked paprika	2 mL
¼ tsp	sea salt	1 mL
¼ tsp	freshly ground black pepper	1 mL
8	slices sourdough bread (½-inch/1 cm thick slices)	8
2 cups	watercress leaves	500 mL

TOPPINGS, OPTIONAL

Avocado slices

Tomato slices

1 Place eggs in a large saucepan and add enough cold water to cover. Bring to a boil over high heat. Remove pan from heat. Cover and let stand for 15 minutes. Fill a medium bowl with 1 quart (1 L) of cold water and ice cubes and transfer eggs to chill for 5 minutes. Peel off shells and finely dice eggs.

2 In a medium bowl, combine eggs, mayonnaise, chives, smoked paprika, salt and pepper. Cover and refrigerate for at least 30 minutes or for up to 2 days to allow flavors to blend and mixture to chill slightly.

3 Lightly toast bread and place on a work surface. Divide egg salad equally among 4 bread slices. Top with watercress, avocados and tomatoes, if desired, and cover with remaining bread.

NUTRIENTS	CALORIES	FAT	CARBOHYDRATE	PROTEIN	FIBER
per serving	950	21.4 g	145.5 g	43 g	6.4 g

How to Build and Bake a Pizza

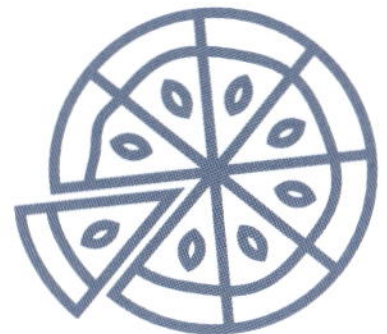

Beyond its ease, homemade pizza is just plain fun. Family members can build their own, and creative cooks can let their imaginations run wild. The same simple method of assembly and construction applies to both these recipes.

To build a pizza, place an 18- by 16-inch (45 by 40 cm) piece of heavy aluminum foil on a work surface. Brush with oil and place the dough in the center.

Flour your hands and spread dough into a rough 14-inch (35 cm) circle, making the circle as thin as you want but leaving a rim at least ½ inch (1 cm) high to contain the filling during baking.

If the dough should tear while you're pushing it into place, pinch it with your fingers to seal it, or patch it with a small scrap of dough.

Arrange the filling on top, as described in the recipes (see facing page), and slide the pizza, still on its foil backing, onto the middle rack of a preheated 450°F (230°C) oven.

Bake for 20 to 25 minutes, or until dough is puffed and crisp.

Remove, slice and serve. Makes 8 small slices, enough for 2 to 3 portions.

See ingredient lists with individual recipes. If you have a favorite recipe for making your own dough, go ahead and use it, but the basis for these recipes is 10 oz (300 g) of thawed, ready-to-bake frozen bread dough.

Follow this method when building the Roasted Eggplant and Feta Pizza (page 150) and the Tomato, Fennel and Olive Pizza (page 151).

Roasted Eggplant and Feta Pizza

MAKES 2 TO 3 SERVINGS

Preheat oven to 450°F (230°C)

TIP
Follow the directions on page 149 to build and bake this pizza.

1	medium to large eggplant	1
3 tbsp	extra-virgin olive oil	45 mL
2	cloves garlic, minced	2
2 tbsp	freshly squeezed lemon juice	30 mL
1 tbsp	chopped fresh Italian (flat-leaf) parsley	15 mL
	Salt and freshly ground black pepper to taste	
10 oz	thawed, ready-to-bake frozen bread dough	300 g
6 oz	feta cheese, crumbled	175 g

Roast eggplant by placing it over a high gas flame or under a broiler until its skin is uniformly blackened. Let cool, slice off stem, peel off skin with your fingers, and dice flesh.

In a large skillet, heat oil over medium-high heat.

Add garlic, eggplant, lemon juice, parsley, salt and pepper; bring to a simmer.

Spread over dough and scatter feta over top.

NUTRIENTS	CALORIES	FAT	CARBOHYDRATE	PROTEIN	FIBER
per serving	636	33.2 g	65.1 g	19.7 g	7.6 g

Tomato, Fennel and Olive Pizza

MAKES 2 TO 3 SERVINGS

Preheat oven to 450°F (230°C)

TIP
Follow the directions on page 149 to build and bake this pizza.

10 oz	thawed, ready-to-bake frozen bread dough	300 g
2 tbsp	olive oil, divided	30 mL
6	plum (Roma) tomatoes, peeled, seeded and coarsely puréed	6
1 cup	diced fennel bulb	250 mL
1 cup	shredded mozzarella cheese	250 mL
1 cup	oil-cured black olives, pitted and coarsely chopped	250 mL
2 tbsp	freshly grated Parmesan cheese	30 mL
Pinch	dried oregano	Pinch
	Salt and freshly ground black pepper to taste	

Brush dough with half the oil.

Spread tomatoes over dough, scatter fennel over tomato, sprinkle evenly with mozzarella, and scatter olives over the cheese.

Sprinkle evenly with Parmesan, oregano, salt and pepper. Drizzle with the remaining oil.

NUTRIENTS	CALORIES	FAT	CARBOHYDRATE	PROTEIN	FIBER
per serving	629	30 g	69 g	22.6 g	7.6 g

Tofu Sandwiches with Tomatoes, Lettuce and Avocado

4	6-inch (15 cm) baguette pieces	4
1	avocado, sliced	1
	Hot pepper sauce	
12	slices Baked Marinated Tofu (page 153)	12
1	tomato, sliced	1
4	leaves romaine lettuce	4
4 tsp	Dijon mustard	20 mL

1 Split baguette pieces in half and tear out some of the center of each to make a trough for the filling.

2 Place avocado slices on bottom halves of baguette and mash lightly. Sprinkle with hot pepper sauce to taste. Cover with tofu, then tomato and romaine. Spread mustard over cut sides of top halves of baguette and close sandwiches.

3 Secure with toothpicks and serve, or wrap tightly and refrigerate overnight.

NUTRIENTS	CALORIES	FAT	CARBOHYDRATE	PROTEIN	FIBER
per serving	420	18.6 g	47.3 g	21 g	6.9 g

Baked Marinated Tofu

This tofu is a versatile prep item, ready to go into sandwiches, stir-fries and other dishes with no frying or extra prep time. The baking time is flexible, depending on both the tofu and your taste (see Tip).

Large square food storage tub (preferably 10 inches/25 cm square)

TIPS

Water-packed tofu comes in varying levels of firmness, from soft to extra-firm. The firmer it is, the more water has been pressed out before it was packaged. Aseptic-packaged tofu is silken tofu, which is too soft for this method. Extra-firm tofu, made with a little extra nigari coagulant and pressed longer, is already so dense that it will be chewy and firm within 40 minutes of baking. If you use standard firm tofu instead, it will be coated and have crispy edges in 40 minutes, but to get a nice, dense texture, give it a full hour.

For a more flavor-infused, chewier tofu, slice the tofu as in Step 1 and freeze it until solid, then thaw in the refrigerator and proceed with Step 2.

2	large rimmed baking sheets, lined with parchment paper	2
24 oz	water-packed extra-firm tofu	750 g
2 tbsp	packed light brown sugar	30 mL
½ tsp	cayenne pepper	2 mL
½ cup	tamari	125 mL
½ cup	unsweetened apple juice	125 mL
2 tbsp	toasted (dark) sesame oil	30 mL

1 Drain tofu and wrap in clean tea towels, pressing gently to remove excess water. Cut each block of tofu into 10 ½-inch (1 cm) slices and place in storage tub.

2 In a small bowl, whisk together brown sugar, cayenne, tamari, apple juice and sesame oil. Pour over tofu. Seal the lid and shake container gently to coat all the slices. Flip container carefully to move marinade between the slices. Refrigerate overnight.

3 Preheat oven to 400°F (200°C).

4 Remove tofu slices from marinade and place on prepared baking sheets, spacing them apart. Drizzle tops with a little marinade. Discard the remaining marinade.

5 Bake for 40 minutes (see Tip), turning tofu slices with a spatula and reversing the positions of the pans halfway through. Let cool completely on pans on wire racks.

6 Transfer cooled tofu to airtight containers and store in the refrigerator for up to 1 week or in the freezer for up to 4 months.

NUTRIENTS	CALORIES	FAT	CARBOHYDRATE	PROTEIN	FIBER
per serving	52	3.2 g	2.8 g	4.2 g	0.4 g

Health Wraps

1 cup	bulgur	250 mL
1½ cups	cold water	375 mL
¼ cup	olive oil	50 mL
3	green onions, finely chopped	3
1	clove garlic, minced	1
1	carrot, shredded	1
1	tomato, chopped	1
2 tbsp	finely chopped fresh mint	30 mL
	Juice of 1 lemon	
6	8-inch (20 cm) whole wheat flour tortillas	6
¾ cup	tahini	175 mL
⅔ cup	alfalfa sprouts	150 mL

Soak bulgur in water and oil for 30 minutes; drain off excess liquid.

Mix in green onions, garlic, carrot, tomato, mint and lemon juice.

In a hot, dry skillet, toast tortillas for 30 seconds per side.

Spread warm tortillas with tahini and top each with a portion of the bulgur mixture. Top with alfalfa sprouts and roll up.

Wrap in waxed paper or parchment, leaving one end open. Eat like pop-up Popsicles.

NUTRIENTS per serving	CALORIES 498	FAT 28.4 g	CARBOHYDRATE 53 g	PROTEIN 13.2 g	FIBER 16.7 g

Gorgonzola Grinders

Preheat oven to 400°F (200°C)

2	cloves garlic, minced	2
½ cup	olive oil	125 mL
⅓ cup	red wine vinegar	75 mL
2 tbsp	chopped fresh basil	30 mL
2 tbsp	chopped fresh chives	30 mL
2 tbsp	chopped fresh Italian (flat-leaf) parsley	30 mL
½ tsp	hot pepper flakes	2 mL
	Freshly ground black pepper to taste	
4	torpedo rolls, split lengthwise	4
1 lb	Gorgonzola cheese, cubed	500 g

Combine garlic, oil, vinegar, basil, chives, parsley, hot pepper flakes and black pepper.

Brush the interior of the rolls with a thin film of this dressing and pack with Gorgonzola.

Pour the remaining dressing over the cheese.

Wrap sandwiches in foil and bake for 10 minutes.

NUTRIENTS per serving	CALORIES	FAT	CARBOHYDRATE	PROTEIN	FIBER
	814	62.1 g	33.5 g	30.2 g	1.5 g

Veggie and Goat Cheese Wraps

4	8-inch (20 cm) tomato basil-flavored flour tortillas, warmed (see Tips)	4
½ cup	hummus	125 mL
1 cup	spring mix greens	250 mL
1 cup	cucumber slices	250 mL
2	tomatoes, thinly sliced	2
1	red bell pepper, cut into thin slices	1
1 cup	alfalfa sprouts	250 mL
½ cup	whole almonds	125 mL
½ cup	green pumpkin seeds (pepitas), toasted	125 mL
4 oz	crumbled goat cheese	125 g

1. Place tortillas on a work surface. Spread 2 tbsp (30 mL) of the hummus down center of tortillas. Arrange greens, cucumber, tomatoes, bell pepper and sprouts over hummus. Top with almonds, pepitas and goat cheese. Fold both edges over filling. Roll up and serve immediately.

Variation

Use feta cheese instead of the goat cheese and whole wheat tortillas instead of tomato basil.

Nuts and Seeds

Nuts and seeds offer great benefits, including an omega-3 boost, antioxidants, magnesium, fiber and health-health fats. They are especially valuable for their potent anti-inflammatory effects.

NUTRIENTS per serving	CALORIES 570	FAT 35.8 g	CARBOHYDRATE 42.4 g	PROTEIN 25.7 g	FIBER 18.1 g

Crispy Baked Falafel

MAKES 4 SERVINGS

Vegetarians and carnivores alike will munch happily on these crispy-perfect falafel. The secret to their success is using soaked dried chickpeas for an ideal texture, and cumin, red onion and fresh herbs for great flavor.

18- by 13-inch (45 by 33 cm) rimmed sheet pan

Food processor

TIPS

Do not substitute canned chickpeas for the soaked dried chickpeas; the texture will be very mushy and the mixture will be too loose to shape into patties.

The patties can be prepared through Step 3, but place them on a sheet pan lined with parchment paper instead of an oiled pan. Freeze until firm, then transfer patties to an airtight container or sealable freezer bag and freeze for up to 3 months. Thaw at room temperature for 2 hours, then bake as directed.

1¼ cups	dried chickpeas	310 mL
4 tbsp	olive oil, divided	60 mL
4	cloves garlic	4
¾ cup	packed fresh flat-leaf (Italian) parsley leaves	175 mL
¾ cup	packed fresh cilantro leaves	175 mL
⅔ cup	coarsely chopped red onion	150 mL
1½ tsp	ground cumin	7 mL
1 tsp	salt	5 mL
½ tsp	freshly ground black pepper	2 mL

SUGGESTED ACCOMPANIMENTS

Warm pita bread

Sliced cucumber

Sliced tomatoes

Fresh spinach, arugula or lettuce leaves

Plain Greek yogurt

Crumbled feta or goat cheese

1. Pick through chickpeas and remove any stones or discolored peas. Place peas in a medium bowl and add enough water to cover by about 2 inches (5 cm). Cover bowl and let soak at room temperature overnight. Drain well.

2. Preheat oven to 375°F (190°C). Pour half the oil onto pan and, using your fingers, spread oil to cover pan.

3. In food processor, combine chickpeas, garlic, parsley, cilantro, onion, cumin, salt, pepper and the remaining oil; process until smooth. Shape into patties that are ½ inch (1 cm) thick and 2 inches (5 cm) in diameter. Place on prepared pan, spacing evenly.

4. Bake in preheated oven for 15 minutes. Open oven door and, using a spatula, carefully turn patties over. Close door and bake for 12 to 15 minutes or until falafel are browned. Serve warm with any of the suggested accompaniments, as desired.

NUTRIENTS	CALORIES	FAT	CARBOHYDRATE	PROTEIN	FIBER
per serving	222	15.4	17.7 g	5.1 g	4.8 g

Warm Italian Wraps

MAKES 4 SERVINGS

If you're in the mood for something Italian, this recipe is great. The roasted vegetables are also fabulous on top of a pizza.

Preheat oven to 450°F (230°C)

Large baking sheet, lightly greased

TIP

I used shredded mozzarella cheese rather than fresh mozzarella packed in brine, because it melts better.

2		eggplants, cut into 1-inch (2.5 cm) pieces	2
3		Roma (plum) tomatoes, thinly sliced	3
1 cup		sliced onion	250 mL
1 cup		sliced red bell pepper	250 mL
1 cup		sliced yellow bell pepper	250 mL
2		cloves garlic, minced	2
1 tbsp		Italian seasoning	15 mL
¼ tsp		hot pepper flakes	1 mL
2 tbsp		balsamic vinegar	30 mL
2 tbsp		olive oil	30 mL
4		8-inch (20 cm) white or whole wheat tortillas	4
4		slices mozzarella cheese	4
2 oz		freshly grated Parmesan cheese	60 g

1. On a prepared baking sheet, arrange eggplant, tomatoes, onion and red and yellow bell peppers. Sprinkle with garlic, Italian seasoning and hot pepper flakes. Drizzle with balsamic vinegar and olive oil. Bake vegetables in preheated oven for 30 minutes or until tender.

2. Place tortillas on a work surface. Arrange vegetables equally in center of each tortilla. Top with mozzarella and Parmesan cheeses. Fold both edges over filling and wrap each filled tortilla in foil. Reduce oven temperature to 325°F (160°C) and bake for 5 minutes or until cheese is melted.

A Rainbow of Veggies

Aiming for a rainbow of colorful vegetables and at least two servings daily can be a great way to manage gout symptoms, increase the amount of daily fiber, decrease hunger and maintain a healthy weight.

NUTRIENTS	CALORIES	FAT	CARBOHYDRATE	PROTEIN	FIBER
per serving	469	20.8 g	55.2 g	19.1 g	21 g

Warm Kale, Tomato and Chickpea Salad

MAKES 4 SERVINGS

Creamy, nutty chickpeas are roasted alongside red onions and tomatoes for this satisfying main-dish salad. A lemony yogurt tahini dressing adds contrasting fresh, bold flavor.

Preheat oven to 400°F (200°C)

18- by 13-inch (45 by 33 cm) rimmed sheet pan, lined with foil or parchment paper

TIPS

You can use 2 cups (500 mL) cherry or grape tomatoes in place of the plum tomatoes.

An equal amount of ground cumin can be used in place of the coriander.

It is best to use regular yogurt, not Greek yogurt, in the sauce; the latter will make the sauce too thick. If Greek yogurt is what you have on hand, use 2 tbsp (30 mL) Greek yogurt plus 2 tbsp (30 mL) water in place of the ¼ cup (60 mL) yogurt.

SALAD

2	cloves garlic, minced	2
1 tsp	ground coriander	5 mL
	Salt and freshly cracked black pepper	
¼ cup	olive oil	60 mL
4	plum (Roma) tomatoes, quartered lengthwise	4
1	large red onion, halved lengthwise and cut crosswise into ¼-inch (0.5 cm) slices	1
2	cans (each 14 to 19 oz/398 to 540 mL) chickpeas, drained and rinsed	2
6 cups	packed chopped kale (tough stems and center ribs removed)	1.5 L

YOGURT TAHINI DRESSING

¼ cup	plain yogurt	60 mL
2 tbsp	well-stirred tahini	30 mL
1½ tbsp	freshly squeezed lemon juice	22 mL
1 tsp	liquid honey or granulated sugar	5 mL

1. **SALAD:** In a small bowl, combine garlic, coriander, ½ tsp (2 mL) salt, ¼ tsp (1 mL) pepper and oil.

2. In a large bowl, toss together tomatoes, onion, chickpeas and half the oil mixture. Spread in a single layer on prepared pan. Roast in preheated oven for 20 to 25 minutes or until tomatoes are softened.

3. In the same large bowl, toss kale with the remaining oil mixture.

4. Open oven door and distribute kale over chickpeas and vegetables. Close door and roast for 8 to 12 minutes or until edges of kale are slightly browned and appear crispy. Let cool on pan for 10 minutes.

5. **DRESSING:** Meanwhile, in a small bowl, whisk together yogurt, tahini, lemon juice and honey. Season to taste with salt and pepper. Drizzle salad with 2 tbsp (30 mL) of the dressing and toss to coat.

6. Divide salad among four dinner plates or shallow dinner bowls. Drizzle with the remaining dressing.

NUTRIENTS	CALORIES	FAT	CARBOHYDRATE	PROTEIN	FIBER
per serving	420	22.3 g	45.5 g	14.3 g	12.5 g

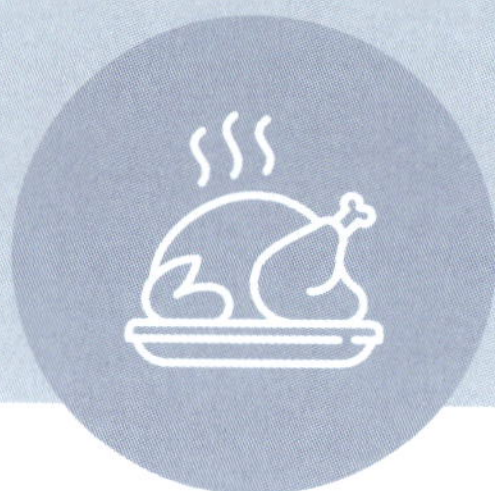

CHAPTER 7

Dinner

Roast Chicken Quarters with Lemon-Dill Spring Vegetables   162

Brined and Tender Lemon Roast Chicken   163

Chicken Florentine with Wild Rice   164

Pasta with Chicken and Vegetable Sauce   165

Chicken Mole   166

Red Enchilada Sauce   167

Chicken and Vegetable Stew   168

Southwestern Shepherd's Pie   169

Pork Tenderloin with Charred Corn Salad   170

Grilled Fish Sandwich   171

Fish and Spinach Tenga   172

Broiled Halibut and Pepper Skewers with Pesto Butter Toasts   173

Roasted Salmon and Root Vegetables with Horseradish Sauce   174

Chili-Glazed Salmon with Brussels Sprouts   175

Lentil-Stuffed Eggplant   176

Legume and Veggie Burgers   178

Tofu and Bok Choy with Gingery Black Beans   179

Chile Tofu and Green Beans   180

Bok Choy, Tofu and Shiitake Stir-Fry   182

Green Pad See Ew   183

Whole Wheat Pasta with Spring Vegetables and Edamame   184

Fettuccine with Fennel and Artichokes   186

Penne with Eggplant and Mushrooms   187

Mushroom-Spinach Lasagna with Goat Cheese   188

Roast Chicken Quarters with Lemon-Dill Spring Vegetables

MAKES 4 SERVINGS

This combination of roasted chicken, fingerling potatoes and spring vegetables is fancy enough for a dinner party but quick and easy enough for a weeknight.

Preheat oven to 500°F (260°C)

18- by 13-inch (45 by 33 cm) rimmed sheet pan, lined with foil

TIP
An equal amount of chopped fresh parsley or mint can be used in place of the dill.

4	chicken leg quarters (about 3 lbs/1.5 kg), patted dry	4
3 tbsp	olive oil, divided	45 mL
	Salt and freshly ground black pepper	
1	package (12 oz/375 g) frozen pearl onions, thawed	1
1	package (1 lb/500 g) peeled baby carrots	1
1 lb	yellow-fleshed fingerling or baby potatoes, halved crosswise	500 g
2 cups	trimmed radishes, halved lengthwise	500 mL
¼ cup	chopped fresh dill	60 mL
1 tbsp	finely grated lemon zest	15 mL
2 tbsp	freshly squeezed lemon juice	30 mL

1. Place chicken, skin side up, on prepared pan, spacing evenly. Brush with 1 tbsp (15 mL) oil and season generously with salt and pepper. Roast in preheated oven for 10 minutes.

2. Meanwhile, in a large bowl, gently toss together onions, carrots, potatoes, radishes, the remaining oil, ¾ tsp (3 mL) salt and ½ tsp (2 mL) pepper.

3. Remove pan from oven and nestle vegetables around the chicken pieces. Roast for 20 to 25 minutes or until vegetables are tender, chicken skin is crispy and an instant-read thermometer inserted in the thickest part of a chicken thigh registers 165°F (74°C).

4. Transfer chicken to a serving platter or individual plates. Sprinkle vegetables with dill, lemon zest and lemon juice, then toss to coat. Serve with chicken.

NUTRIENTS	CALORIES	FAT	CARBOHYDRATE	PROTEIN	FIBER
per serving	993	64.8 g	40.1 g	60.5 g	7.7 g

Brined and Tender Lemon Roast Chicken

Joanne says that if she takes the entire chicken to the table, it will all be eaten. But if she presents a dinner plate with the chicken already portioned, everyone eats less and the remaining chicken can be served at another meal.

TIPS

Brining chicken in a mild salt solution produces delightfully tender meat. Do not brine the chicken for longer than 8 hours. Over-brining may adversely affect the texture of the cooked chicken.

Tenting the chicken with foil and letting it rest before carving allows the juices to redistribute throughout the meat, creating a much moister chicken.

Joanne Rankin, Dietitian, British Columbia

1	whole roasting chicken (3 to 4 lbs/1.5 to 2 kg)	1
3 tbsp	kosher salt	45 mL
12 cups	water	3 L
1	lemon	1
2 tsp	canola or olive oil	10 mL
½ tsp	salt	2 mL

1. Trim excess fat from chicken. Rinse inside and out under cold running water.

2. In a large pot, combine kosher salt and water, stirring to dissolve salt. Add chicken, breast side down, making sure it is fully submerged. Cover and refrigerate for at least 4 hours or for up to 8 hours.

3. About 30 minutes before cooking, drain brine from chicken and discard. Rinse chicken under running water and pat dry. Place on a clean plate and let stand at room temperature.

4. Place oven rack in center of oven, place empty roasting pan on rack and preheat oven to 425°F (220°C).

5. Meanwhile, place whole lemon in a small saucepan and add water to cover. Bring to a boil over high heat. Reduce heat and simmer for 5 minutes. Remove from heat and leave lemon in hot water until ready to use.

6. Rub chicken all over with oil and sprinkle with ½ tsp (2 mL) salt. Remove the lemon from the hot water, discarding water. Poke several holes in the lemon and insert it into the cavity of the chicken.

7. Carefully remove the hot roasting pan from the oven, place chicken, breast side up, in pan, and roast for 30 minutes. Reduce heat to 400°F (200°C). Roast chicken for 60 minutes or until skin is dark golden and crispy, drumsticks wiggle when touched and a meat thermometer inserted in the thickest part of a thigh registers 185°F (85°C). Transfer chicken to a cutting board, tent with foil and let rest for 10 to 15 minutes before carving.

8. Using kitchen tongs, remove lemon from the chicken. Cut lemon in half and squeeze juice over hot chicken pieces.

Variation

For added flavor, insert fresh or dried herbs, such as thyme, rosemary, savory or marjoram, into the cavity of the chicken along with the lemon.

NUTRIENTS	CALORIES	FAT	CARBOHYDRATE	PROTEIN	FIBER
per serving	168	7.6 g	1 g	23 g	0 g

Chicken Florentine with Wild Rice

MAKES 4 SERVINGS

This beautiful dish features layers of long-grain and wild rice, chicken and spinach, covered with a fabulous cheesy, creamy sauce.

Preheat oven to 375°F (190°C)

13- by 9-inch (33 by 23 cm) glass baking dish, greased

TIPS

White rice works beautifully in this recipe in place of the long-grain and wild rice blend. Cook white rice according to package instructions before adding it to the baking dish in Step 6.

If you like sharp cheese, use extra-sharp (extra-old) Cheddar.

When you're assembling the casserole, the spinach will fill the dish and be slightly mounded. You may need to press it down a little to keep it from falling out, but it will wilt quickly in the oven, so you don't have to worry about the dish overflowing.

1 cup	long-grain and wild rice blend (6 oz/175 g)	250 mL
¼ cup	all-purpose flour	60 mL
½ tsp	salt	2 mL
½ tsp	freshly ground black pepper	2 mL
4	boneless skinless chicken breasts	4
1 tbsp	all-purpose flour	15 mL
1 tbsp	olive oil	15 mL
1 tbsp	butter	15 mL
¼ cup	dry white wine	60 mL
½ cup	chicken broth	125 mL
½ cup	milk	125 mL
1 cup	shredded Cheddar cheese, divided	250 mL
1	bag (10 oz/300 g) fresh spinach, stems removed	1

1 In a medium saucepan, bring 2¼ cups (550 mL) water to a boil over high heat. Stir in rice mix, reduce heat to low, cover and simmer for 25 minutes or until rice is tender and most of the liquid is absorbed. Remove from heat and let stand, covered, for 5 minutes. Fluff with a fork. Set aside.

2 Meanwhile, in a medium bowl, combine ¼ cup (60 mL) flour, salt and pepper. Dredge chicken in seasoned flour, coating evenly and shaking off excess. Discard excess flour mixture.

3 In a large skillet, heat oil and butter over medium-high heat. Cook chicken, turning once, for about 8 minutes or until browned on both sides. Transfer chicken to a plate.

4 Stir 1 tbsp (15 mL) flour into fat remaining in skillet and cook, stirring constantly, for 1 minute. Reduce heat to low and gradually stir in wine, broth and milk, scraping up any brown bits from bottom of pan. Simmer, stirring constantly, until thick and bubbling. Add ¾ cup (175 mL) of the cheese, stirring until melted. Remove from heat and set aside.

5 Spoon cooked rice into prepared baking dish. Place chicken on top and cover with spinach. Pour cheese sauce over top and sprinkle with the remaining ¼ cup (60 mL) cheese.

6 Bake in preheated oven for 30 minutes or until chicken is no longer pink inside.

NUTRIENTS	CALORIES	FAT	CARBOHYDRATE	PROTEIN	FIBER
per serving	613	21.4 g	47.9 g	51.9 g	3.1 g

Pasta with Chicken and Vegetable Sauce

MAKES 8 SERVINGS

Leftover chicken takes on a new life in this delicious pasta sauce.

TIPS

Cold chicken shredded by hand into irregular, bite-size pieces is more visually appealing and creates more surface area for the flavorful sauce to cling to than cubes cut with a knife.

For the best texture, be careful not to boil the chicken in the sauce.

If your family is just starting to eat whole wheat pasta, mix it half and half with regular pasta at first. Gradually increase the percentage of whole wheat until the whole dish is whole-grain.

Joanne Rankin, Dietitian, British Columbia

1 lb	whole wheat penne or rotini pasta	500 g
2 tbsp	canola or olive oil	30 mL
1 cup	chopped onion	250 mL
3	cloves garlic, minced	3
½ tsp	hot pepper flakes (optional)	2 mL
4 cups	bite-size broccoli florets (about 1 large head)	1 L
1 cup	canned diced tomatoes with juice	250 mL
1½ cups	shredded cooked chicken	375 mL
2 tbsp	basil pesto	30 mL
½ cup	coarsely chopped fresh parsley	125 mL
¼ tsp	salt	1 mL
	Freshly ground black pepper	
½ cup	freshly grated Parmesan cheese	125 mL

1. In a large pot of boiling salted water, cook pasta according to package directions until al dente. Drain, reserving ½ cup (125 mL) of the cooking water. Transfer pasta to a large serving bowl.

2. Meanwhile, in a large skillet, heat oil over medium-high heat. Sauté onion for about 3 minutes or until softened and edges are lightly browned. Add garlic and hot pepper flakes (if using); sauté for 30 seconds. Add broccoli and cook, stirring occasionally, for about 5 minutes or until bright green.

3. Stir in tomatoes and bring to a boil. Stir in chicken, pesto and reserved pasta water. Reduce heat and simmer, stirring often, for about 3 minutes or until chicken is heated through. Remove from heat and stir in parsley, salt and pepper to taste.

4. Pour sauce over pasta and stir to combine. Sprinkle with Parmesan.

Variation

Use leftover turkey or meatballs instead of chicken.

NUTRIENTS	CALORIES	FAT	CARBOHYDRATE	PROTEIN	FIBER
per serving	347	9.5 g	49 g	20 g	6 g

Chicken Mole

Chicken served with a richly flavored sauce is popular in many parts of Mexico. The earthy, sweet flavor of the sauce defines this dish.

Preheat oven to 350°F (180°C)

13- by 9-inch (33 by 23 cm) casserole dish, greased

TIP
Add a pinch of cinnamon and ½ tsp (2 mL) granulated sugar to the sauce with the spices for a sweeter version. Sprinkle finished dish with toasted sesame seeds.

2 cups	Red Enchilada Sauce (page 167)	500 mL
1 tsp	hot pepper flakes	5 mL
1 tsp	dried oregano	5 mL
1 tsp	ground cumin	5 mL
1 tsp	garlic powder	5 mL
1 tsp	onion powder	5 mL
1½ oz	semisweet chocolate, chopped into small pieces	45 g
3 tbsp	olive oil	45 mL
4- to 5-lb	whole chicken, cut into 8 pieces	2 to 2.5 kg
	Salt and freshly ground black pepper	

1 In a saucepan, heat sauce over medium heat until bubbly. Stir in hot pepper flakes, oregano, cumin, garlic powder and onion powder. Reduce heat and simmer, stirring often, until flavors are blended, 3 to 5 minutes. Reduce heat to low and stir in chocolate until melted. Set aside.

2 In a large pot, heat oil over medium-high heat. Add chicken pieces, in batches to avoid crowding, and brown, turning once, for 3 to 4 minutes per side. Lightly season with salt and pepper. Transfer to prepared casserole dish. Repeat with remaining chicken, adjusting heat as necessary between batches.

3 Spread sauce evenly over chicken. Bake in preheated oven until juices run clear when chicken is pierced, about 45 minutes. Serve immediately.

NUTRIENTS	CALORIES	FAT	CARBOHYDRATE	PROTEIN	FIBER
per serving	713	55.2 g	17.8 g	36.5 g	4.2 g

Red Enchilada Sauce

MAKES 2 CUPS (500 ML)

SERVING SIZE: 2 TBSP (30 ML)

This authentic sauce is traditional in some regions of the Southwest. Made from dried red chiles, it is a time-consuming process but worth the effort. Dried New Mexico red chile peppers are generally 4 to 6 inches (10 to 15 cm) in length. They can be found in the produce department or Mexican food section.

Blender or food processor

6 to 8	dried New Mexico red chile peppers	6 to 8
6 tbsp	vegetable oil, divided	90 mL
4	cloves garlic, minced	4
2 tbsp	all-purpose flour	30 mL
	Kosher salt and freshly ground black pepper	

1. Place chiles in a bowl and cover with 1 quart (1 L) of water. Refrigerate overnight. This will soften the chiles.

2. Drain soaking liquid from chiles, reserving liquid. In a blender, purée chiles with 1½ cups (375 mL) reserved liquid until smooth. Purée should be thick but pourable. Add additional soaking liquid, if needed. Press chile purée through a fine-mesh sieve or a strainer, discarding skin and seeds.

3. In a large skillet, heat 2 tbsp (30 mL) of the oil over medium heat. Add chile purée and garlic. Bring to a gentle boil. Reduce heat to low and simmer, stirring occasionally, until flavors are well blended, 8 to 10 minutes. Set aside.

4. In a small saucepan, heat remaining ¼ cup (60 mL) of oil over medium heat. Gradually stir in flour, creating a roux (a thick paste). Remove from heat.

5. Increase heat to medium. Gradually stir roux into chile sauce. Reduce heat and simmer, stirring, until thick and smooth, 6 to 8 minutes. Season with salt and pepper to taste. Serve immediately or let cool to room temperature. Transfer to an airtight container and refrigerate for up to 2 days.

NUTRIENTS per serving	CALORIES	FAT	CARBOHYDRATE	PROTEIN	FIBER
	61	5.3 g	3.4 g	0.5 g	1 g

Chicken and Vegetable Stew

MAKES 4 SERVINGS

SERVING SIZE:
1½ CUPS (375 ML)

One of the easiest
ways to use up extra
frozen vegetables
is to add them to
dishes like this stew.
It's also an easy way
to help you reach
your daily dose of
vegetables—adding
fresh, frozen or
canned varieties can
help meet your needs.

TIP
To lessen cooking time,
use leftover baked russet
or sweet potatoes and
add as directed in Step 1.
Reduce the simmer time
to 10 minutes, instead of
20 minutes.

1 tbsp	olive oil or canola oil	15 mL
1	yellow onion, chopped	1
2	cloves garlic, minced	2
3 tbsp	all-purpose flour	45 mL
1 tsp	dried thyme	5 mL
½ tsp	dried basil	2 mL
3 cups	shredded rotisserie chicken	750 mL
2 cups	reduced-sodium ready-to-use chicken broth	500 mL
2 russet	potatoes, diced into 1-inch (2.5 cm) cubes	2
3	carrots, cut into 1-inch (2.5 cm) rounds	3
1	red bell pepper, cut into 1-inch (2.5 cm) strips	1
1 cup	frozen peas	250 mL
¼ cup	white cooking wine or dry white wine	60 mL
3	bay leaves	3
¼ tsp	salt	1 mL
¼ tsp	freshly ground black pepper	1 mL

1 In a large stockpot, heat the oil over medium heat. When the oil is shimmering, add the onion and garlic and cook, stirring occasionally, until the onion is translucent and the garlic is fragrant, about 2 minutes. Sprinkle in the flour, thyme and basil and stir for 2 minutes. Add the chicken, broth, potatoes, carrots, red pepper, peas, wine, bay leaves, salt and pepper. Raise the heat to high and bring the mixture to a boil. Reduce the heat to medium-low and simmer, covered, for 20 minutes. Remove the bay leaves before serving.

NUTRIENTS	CALORIES	FAT	CARBOHYDRATE	PROTEIN	FIBER
per serving	407	11.2 g	41 g	33.1 g	7.3 g

Southwestern Shepherd's Pie

MAKES 6 SERVINGS

Traditional shepherd's pie is great, but shepherd's pie with a little kick of the Southwest? Terrific!

Preheat oven to 350°F (180°C)

11- by 7-inch (28 by 18 cm) glass baking dish

1½ lbs	Yukon gold potatoes, cut into 1-inch (2.5 cm) cubes	750 g
½ cup	milk	125 mL
2 tbsp	butter	30 mL
2 tbsp	chopped fresh cilantro	30 mL
1 tsp	salt, divided	5 mL
1 tsp	freshly ground black pepper, divided	5 mL
1 lb	lean ground beef	500 g
2	cloves garlic, minced	2
½ cup	chopped onion	125 mL
1	can (14 to 19 oz/398 to 540 mL) black beans, drained and rinsed	1
1	can (14 oz/398 mL) diced tomatoes	1
1½ cups	corn kernels (thawed if frozen)	375 mL
½ cup	shredded Cheddar cheese	125 mL

1. Place potatoes in a large saucepan and add enough water to cover. Cover and bring to a boil over high heat. Reduce heat and simmer for about 15 minutes or until potatoes are just tender. Drain, return to the pot and add milk, butter, cilantro, half the salt and half the pepper; mash until smooth.

2. Meanwhile, in a large nonstick skillet, over medium-high heat, cook beef, garlic and onion, breaking beef up with the back of a spoon, for 8 to 10 minutes or until beef is no longer pink. Drain off fat.

3. Stir in beans, tomatoes and the remaining salt and pepper; bring to a boil. Reduce heat and simmer, stirring often, for 5 to 7 minutes or until heated through.

4. Spread beef mixture in baking dish. Spread corn evenly over meat. Spread mashed potatoes over corn. Sprinkle with cheese.

5. Bake in preheated oven for 20 minutes or until top is golden.

NUTRIENTS per serving	CALORIES 514	FAT 15.1 g	CARBOHYDRATE 67 g	PROTEIN 29.6 g	FIBER 11.6 g

Pork Tenderloin with Charred Corn Salad

MAKES 4 SERVINGS

Pork tenderloin is terrific for showcasing any number of flavors, but don't think you need to add them all at once. A simple rub of cumin, salt and pepper, for example, is outstanding. The charred corn salad alongside is based on the Mexican corn dish esquites. The word esquites comes from the Nahuatl word ìzquitl, which means "toasted corn," and the dish is a popular street food throughout Mexico. In place of the typical creamy cheese sauce, this version gets a crumble of queso fresco.

Preheat oven to 400°F (200°C)

18- by 13-inch (45 by 33 cm) rimmed sheet pan, lined with parchment paper or foil and sprayed with nonstick cooking spray

TIPS

It will take about 4 to 5 large ears of corn to yield 3 cups (750 mL) corn kernels.

1 lb	pork tenderloin, trimmed and patted dry	500 g
2 tbsp	vegetable oil, divided	30 mL
1 tsp	ground cumin	5 mL
	Salt and freshly cracked black pepper	
3 cups	fresh corn kernels (see Tips)	750 mL
1 tsp	chipotle chile powder	5 mL
2	green onions, thinly sliced	2
1	Hass avocado, diced	1
½ cup	packed fresh cilantro leaves, chopped	125 mL
2 tbsp	crumbled queso fresco or mild feta cheese	30 mL
1 tbsp	freshly squeezed lime juice	15 mL

1 Cut six 1-inch (2.5 cm) slits, evenly spaced, across the top of the tenderloin. Place on prepared pan. Brush with half the oil and sprinkle with cumin, ¼ tsp (1 mL) salt and ¼ tsp (1 mL) pepper. Using your hands, work the seasoning all over the tenderloin.

2 In a large bowl, toss corn with the remaining oil and chile powder. Season with salt and pepper. Spread in a single layer around pork.

3 Roast in preheated oven for 25 to 28 minutes or until corn is browned at edges and an instant-read thermometer inserted in the thickest part of the tenderloin registers 145°F (63°C) for medium-rare.

4 Transfer pork to cutting board and let rest for 5 to 10 minutes before slicing against the grain. Just before serving, add green onions, avocado, cilantro, queso fresco and lime juice to corn on pan, gently tossing to coat. Season to taste with salt and pepper.

Variations

If fresh corn is out of season, use an equal amount of thawed frozen corn kernels. Thoroughly pat the kernels dry with paper towels before roasting.

An equal amount of cumin or regular chili powder, plus ⅛ tsp (0.5 mL) cayenne pepper, can be used in place of the chipotle chile powder.

NUTRIENTS	CALORIES	FAT	CARBOHYDRATE	PROTEIN	FIBER
per serving	745	24 g	99.5 g	37.9 g	13.6 g

Grilled Fish Sandwich

MAKES 4 SERVINGS

Preheat barbecue grill to medium, lightly greased

Grill rack or basket

TIP
Grill fish over medium or medium-low heat. Fish cooks quickly, and you don't want it to overcook.

4	skinless fish fillets, such as grouper, snapper or cod, each about ¾ inch (2 cm) thick (about 2 lbs/1 kg total)	4
1 tsp	lemon pepper	5 mL
1 tsp	sea salt	5 mL
¼ cup	freshly squeezed lemon juice	60 mL
4	whole wheat buns, split and toasted	4

TOPPINGS, OPTIONAL

Prepared cocktail or tartar sauce

Lettuce

Tomato slices

Red onion slices

1 Place fish in a shallow dish. Sprinkle with lemon pepper and salt and drizzle with lemon juice.

2 Grill on grill rack or basket, covered, for 8 minutes per side or until fish flakes easily when tested with a fork.

3 Place buns on a work surface. Place fish on buns and add cocktail sauce, lettuce, tomatoes and onions, as desired.

NUTRIENTS per serving	CALORIES 313	FAT 3.3 g	CARBOHYDRATE 23.5 g	PROTEIN 44.8 g	FIBER 1.0 g

Fish and Spinach Tenga

MAKES 3 TO 4 SERVINGS

Tenga is a slightly sour, broth-like Assamese dish, minimally spiced but surprisingly flavorful. It is served with plain rice.

TIP

Mustard oil is made from cold-pressed mustard seeds and is not an infusion. It has a distinctive taste and is the preferred oil in Bengal and other eastern states. However, it has an element that can be toxic to some. Heating it to smoking point neutralizes this and makes it safe for cooking.

1 lb	skinless fish fillets, such as catfish, snapper, tilapia or cod	500 g
1¼ tsp	salt, divided	6 mL
1 tsp	turmeric	5 mL
¼ cup	mustard oil	50 mL
1 tsp	fenugreek seeds (methi)	5 mL
12 oz to 1 lb	fresh spinach, coarsely chopped	375 to 500 g
2 tbsp	freshly squeezed lime or lemon juice	30 mL

1 Rinse fish and pat dry thoroughly. Cut into 3- to 4-inch (7.5 to 10 cm) pieces.

2 In a bowl, mix together 1 tsp (5 mL) salt and turmeric. Add fish and coat all over with mixture. Set aside for 15 minutes at room temperature or for up to 2 hours in refrigerator.

3 In a wide saucepan, heat oil over high heat until smoking. Remove from heat and let cool for 1 minute (see Tip). Return to medium heat. Add fish and sauté for 2 minutes. Flip pieces and cook just until opaque but not cooked through. Using a slotted spoon, transfer fish to a dish, draining off all but 1 tbsp (15 mL) of the oil.

4 Return saucepan to medium heat. Add fenugreek and sauté for 10 seconds. Add spinach and sauté until spinach is wilted.

5 Add 1 cup (250 mL) water and remaining salt. Bring to a gentle boil. Add fish to pan along with any accumulated juices. Return to a gentle boil. Reduce heat to medium-low, cover and cook until fish flakes easily with tip of knife. Add lime juice. Serve hot with steamed rice.

NUTRIENTS	CALORIES	FAT	CARBOHYDRATE	PROTEIN	FIBER
per serving	282	17.1 g	0.5 g	27.2 g	3.3 g

Broiled Halibut and Pepper Skewers with Pesto Butter Toasts

MAKES 4 SERVINGS

Prepared basil pesto elevates simple preparations like these halibut and bell pepper skewers. It also creates an instant compound butter for rustic bread, which toasts alongside.

Preheat broiler

Four 12-inch (30 cm) metal skewers

18- by 13-inch (45 by 33 cm) rimmed sheet pan, lined with foil and sprayed with nonstick cooking spray

TIP
Sea bass, cod or any other firm white fish fillets may be used in place of the halibut.

1½ lbs	skinless halibut fillet, patted dry and cut into 1-inch (2.5 cm) pieces	750 g
2	red bell peppers, cut into 1-inch (2.5 cm) pieces	2
5 tbsp	basil pesto, divided	75 mL
2 tbsp	white wine vinegar	30 mL
2 tbsp	unsalted butter, softened	30 mL
4	thick slices rustic-style bread	4
½ tsp	salt	2 mL

1 Place fish and red pepper in a shallow dish. Drizzle with 3 tbsp (45 mL) pesto and vinegar, then toss to coat. Let stand for 5 minutes.

2 Meanwhile, in a small bowl, stir together butter and the remaining pesto until blended. Spread on one side of each bread slice.

3 Alternately thread fish and pepper pieces onto skewers, discarding any excess marinade. Place on one side of prepared pan and season with salt.

4 Broil for 6 minutes. Open oven door and turn skewers over. Place bread, buttered side up, on opposite side of pan. Close door and broil for 2 to 3 minutes or until bread is golden brown and fish is opaque and flakes easily when tested with a fork.

Bell Peppers

Bell peppers are a powerhouse of vitamin C. A cup of bell peppers provides more than 200% of your daily vitamin C needs. Here are some vegetables and their typical vitamin C content per 100 grams:

- **Red bell peppers:** 128 mg
- **Green bell peppers:** 80 mg
- **Kale:** 120 mg
- **Broccoli:** 89 mg
- **Brussels sprouts:** 85 mg
- **Spinach:** 28 mg
- **Parsley:** 133 mg

NUTRIENTS per serving	CALORIES	FAT	CARBOHYDRATE	PROTEIN	FIBER
	543	37.7 g	20 g	30.1 g	4 g

Roasted Salmon and Root Vegetables with Horseradish Sauce

MAKES 4 SERVINGS

Sour cream seasoned with horseradish and dill makes a quick and tasty sauce for roasted salmon and root vegetables in this Eastern European–inspired meal.

Preheat oven to 425°F (220°C)

18- by 13-inch (45 by 33 cm) rimmed sheet pan, lined with foil

NUTRITION TIP

For a lighter dish, substitute an equal amount of plain Greek yogurt for the sour cream.

6	carrots, trimmed and cut into ½-inch (1 cm) thick slices	6
4	parsnips, trimmed and cut into ½-inch (1 cm) thick slices	4
4	beets, trimmed and cut into ½-inch (1 cm) thick slices	4
3 tbsp	olive oil, divided	45 mL
	Salt and freshly cracked black pepper	
1 tsp	dried dillweed	5 mL
½ cup	sour cream	125 mL
3 tbsp	prepared horseradish	45 mL
2 tsp	cider vinegar	10 mL
4	pieces (each 6 oz /175 g) skinless salmon fillet, patted dry	4

1 On prepared pan, toss together carrots, parsnips, beets, 2 tbsp (30 mL) oil, ½ tsp (2 mL) salt and ¼ tsp (1 mL) pepper. Spread in a single layer. Roast in preheated oven for 25 minutes.

2 Meanwhile, in a small cup, combine dill, sour cream, horseradish and vinegar until blended. Season to taste with salt and pepper.

3 Remove pan from oven and nestle fish among the vegetables, spacing evenly. Brush fish with the remaining oil and season with salt and pepper. Roast for 9 to 14 minutes or until vegetables are fork-tender and fish is opaque and flakes easily when tested with a fork. Serve with horseradish sauce.

NUTRIENTS	CALORIES	FAT	CARBOHYDRATE	PROTEIN	FIBER
per serving	524	23.9 g	39.2 g	39.2 g	10.7 g

Chili-Glazed Salmon with Brussels Sprouts

MAKES 4 SERVINGS

Honey, chili powder and Dijon mustard create a luscious glaze for roasted salmon. Add oven-caramelized Brussels sprouts and dinner is done!

Preheat oven to 425°F (220°C)

18- by 13-inch (45 by 33 cm) rimmed sheet pan, lined with foil and sprayed with nonstick cooking spray

TIP

An equal amount of agave nectar, pure maple syrup or packed light brown sugar can be used in place of the honey.

1 lb	Brussels sprouts, trimmed and halved lengthwise if large	500 g
3 tbsp	olive oil, divided	45 mL
¾ tsp	salt, divided	3 mL
1½ tsp	chili powder	7 mL
1 tbsp	liquid honey	15 mL
2 tsp	Dijon mustard	10 mL
4	pieces (each 6 oz/175 g) skinless salmon fillet, patted dry	4

1. On prepared pan, toss Brussels sprouts with 2 tbsp (30 mL) oil and ½ tsp (2 mL) salt. Spread in a single layer. Roast in preheated oven for 20 minutes.

2. Meanwhile, in a small cup, combine chili powder, the remaining salt, the remaining oil, honey and mustard.

3. Remove pan from oven and nestle fish among the Brussels sprouts, spacing evenly. Brush fish generously with mustard glaze. Roast for 9 to 14 minutes or until Brussels sprouts are browned and fish is opaque and flakes easily when tested with a fork.

NUTRIENTS	CALORIES	FAT	CARBOHYDRATE	PROTEIN	FIBER
per serving	375	18.2 g	15.1 g	39 g	4.7 g

Lentil-Stuffed Eggplant

SERVING SIZE:
1 EGGPLANT HALF

This nicely portioned main provides a healthy amount of plant-based protein from the lentils, and the canned tomatoes add more immune-boosting benefits with a boatload of the antioxidant vitamin C. Perfect for a meatless dinner any night of the week!

Preheat oven to 400°F (200°C)

Baking sheet coated with cooking spray

Blender or food processor

TIPS

To make this dish gluten-free, use gluten-free panko.

To make this dish vegan, swap nutritional yeast for the Parmesan cheese.

2	eggplants, halved lengthwise	2
¼ cup	olive oil	60 mL
	Salt	
1	yellow onion, chopped	1
1	carrot, chopped	1
2	cloves garlic, minced	2
1	can (14 to 19 oz/398 to 540 mL) low-sodium brown lentils, drained and rinsed	1
1	can (14 oz/398 mL) finely diced tomatoes, with juice	1
1	zucchini, grated	1
½ cup	low-sodium vegetable broth	125 mL
1 tsp	dried parsley flakes	5 mL
½ tsp	smoked paprika	2 mL
⅛ tsp	ground black pepper	0.5 mL
½ cup	grated Parmesan cheese	125 mL
¼ cup	panko bread crumbs, preferably whole wheat	60 mL

1. Scoop out some of the flesh from the eggplant halves, leaving about 1 inch (2.5 cm) around the edge. Set the halves aside.

2. Add the scooped-out flesh and 1 tbsp (15 mL) of the oil to a blender or food processor and purée. Transfer the mixture to a clean bowl and set aside.

3. Brush both sides of the eggplant halves with 1 tbsp (15 mL) of the oil and place on the prepared baking sheet skin side down. Sprinkle ¼ tsp (1 mL) of the salt onto the flesh side of the eggplant halves. Bake until the eggplants are slightly softened and browned, 20 minutes.

4. Reduce the oven temperature to 350°F (180°C).

5. In a large skillet, heat the remaining 2 tbsp (30 mL) oil over medium heat. When the oil is shimmering, add the onion, carrot, and garlic and cook, stirring occasionally, until softened, 5 minutes. Add the puréed eggplant, lentils, tomatoes with juice, zucchini, vegetable broth, parsley, paprika, black pepper and ¼ tsp (1 mL) salt and stir to combine. Increase the heat to high and bring the mixture to a boil. Reduce the heat to medium-low and simmer, stirring occasionally, until the flavors combine, 10 minutes. Remove the skillet from the heat and let cool for 10 minutes.

NUTRIENTS per serving	CALORIES 400	FAT 18.4 g	CARBOHYDRATE 47 g	PROTEIN 17.2 g	FIBER 18.4 g

6 In a small bowl, mix the Parmesan cheese with the panko bread crumbs.

7 Divide the lentil mixture equally between each of the 4 eggplant halves. Top each eggplant half with 3 tbsp (45 mL) of the cheese-panko mixture. Return to the oven and bake until the cheese has melted and the top is slightly browned, 10 minutes. Remove from the oven and let the eggplant cool for 10 minutes.

8 On each of four plates, place 1 eggplant half. Serve warm.

Canned Tomatoes: A Pantry Essential

Canned tomatoes are convenient to use and have a longer shelf life than fresh tomatoes, making them a practical choice for busy lifestyles. Most of the time, canned tomatoes are processed shortly after harvesting, which helps retain their nutritional value. You may use them in various dishes, such as soups, stews, sauces and casseroles.

Tips for Using Canned Tomatoes:
- Look for canned tomatoes with no added salt or sugar to avoid excessive sodium and sweeteners.
- Consider using diced or crushed canned tomatoes for convenience, or whole canned tomatoes for a chunkier texture.
- Drain and rinse canned tomatoes to reduce the sodium content before using them in recipes.
- Store any leftover canned tomatoes in an airtight container in the refrigerator for up to 3 to 4 days or freeze them for longer storage.

Legume and Veggie Burgers

MAKES 6 PATTIES

SERVING SIZE: 1 PATTY

Our recipe testers served these veggie burgers to university students for lunch one day, and they all raved about them—now there's a compliment!

TIPS

Make sure the mushrooms, onion and pepper are finely chopped so that patties stick together.

Choose mild, medium or hot salsa, depending on how much heat you like.

To reduce the sodium, choose buns with the lowest % DV for sodium.

NUTRITION TIP

Rinsing canned beans well under cold water before use both reduces the sodium and, as a bonus, reduces the chance that you will experience uncomfortable and potentially embarrassing gas.

Heather McColl,
Dietitian, British
Columbia

1	can (14 oz/398 mL) red kidney beans, rinsed and drained	1
2	cloves garlic, minced	2
1	carrot, grated	1
½ cup	finely chopped mushrooms	125 mL
½ cup	finely chopped onion	125 mL
½ cup	finely chopped red bell pepper	125 mL
½ cup	quick-cooking rolled oats	125 mL
2 tbsp	salsa	30 mL
¼ tsp	freshly ground black pepper	1 mL
	Vegetable cooking spray	
6	slices (each 1 oz/30 g) Monterey Jack cheese or vegan alternative	6
6	whole-grain buns, split	6

1 In a large bowl, using a fork, mash beans to a coarse texture. Add garlic, carrot, mushrooms, onion, red pepper, oats, salsa and pepper; mix well to combine. Shape into 6 ½-inch (1 cm) thick patties. Place on a large plate and refrigerate for 30 minutes.

2 Spray a nonstick skillet with cooking spray and preheat over medium heat. In batches as necessary, fry patties for 5 to 6 minutes or until bottom is golden. Flip over and fry for 5 to 6 minutes or until bottom is golden and patties are heated through.

3 Top patties with cheese and serve on buns.

NUTRIENTS per serving	CALORIES 409	FAT 13 g	CARBOHYDRATE 54 g	PROTEIN 19 g	FIBER 9 g

Tofu and Bok Choy with Gingery Black Beans

Tofu delivers the pungent flavor of Cantonese-style black bean sauce in this zesty dish.

TIPS

To make soft tofu into firm, drain well and place tofu block on a dinner plate in the sink. Place a second dinner plate on top of tofu. Press down gently on top plate to compress tofu and extract liquid. Tip plates so that liquid drains away. Transfer pressed tofu to a cutting board and pat dry with paper towels or kitchen towels. Cut tofu into ½-inch (1 cm) cubes.

To mash the black beans, ginger and garlic, you could also pile them up on your cutting board and chop them together to blend them into a coarse paste.

2 tbsp	salted black beans	30 mL
2 tbsp	chopped fresh gingerroot	30 mL
2 tsp	chopped garlic	10 mL
¼ cup	vegetable stock or water	60 mL
2 tbsp	dry sherry or Shaoxing rice wine	30 mL
1 tbsp	soy sauce	15 mL
2 tsp	cornstarch	10 mL
½ tsp	granulated sugar	2 mL
2 tbsp	vegetable oil	30 mL
¼ cup	chopped onion	60 mL
4 cups	chopped bok choy (2-inch/5 cm pieces)	1 L
16 oz	firm or extra-firm tofu, drained and cut into ½-inch (1 cm) cubes (see Tips)	500 g
2 tbsp	chopped green onions	30 mL
1 tsp	Asian sesame oil	5 mL

1 In a small bowl, combine black beans, ginger and garlic. Using the back of a spoon, mash everything together to make a rough paste (see Tips). In another small bowl, combine vegetable stock, sherry, soy sauce, cornstarch and sugar and stir well into a smooth sauce. Set both aside.

2 Heat a wok or a large deep skillet over high heat. Add oil and swirl to coat pan. Add onion and toss well, until fragrant and softened, about 15 seconds.

3 Add bok choy and cook, tossing often, until it begins to wilt, about 30 seconds. Add tofu and toss well.

4 Scrape black bean mixture onto bok choy and tofu and toss well. Stir vegetable stock mixture and add to pan, pouring in around sides. Toss well. Cook, tossing occasionally, until bok choy is tender-crisp and tofu is evenly seasoned with sauce, about 2 minutes. (Add 1 to 2 tbsp [15 to 25 mL] of water if needed to keep from burning or sticking to pan.)

5 Add green onions and sesame oil and toss well. Transfer to a serving plate. Serve hot or warm.

NUTRIENTS	CALORIES	FAT	CARBOHYDRATE	PROTEIN	FIBER
per serving	212	14.1 g	9.4 g	13.7 g	2.7 g

Chile Tofu and Green Beans

MAKES 4 SERVINGS

SERVING SIZE: 2 CUPS (500 ML)

You can easily switch up the non-starchy vegetables in this recipe to minimize food waste in your kitchen.

TIP

This recipe calls for steaming the green beans, which keeps the vegetables crisp when cooked. Other firm vegetables that steam well include broccoli, cauliflower and carrots.

2 tbsp plus 2 tsp	olive oil or canola oil, divided	40 mL
1 lb	extra-firm tofu, cut into 1-inch (2.5 cm) cubes	500 g
12 oz	green beans, trimmed	375 g
¼ cup	low-sodium vegetable broth	60 mL
2 tbsp	reduced-sodium soy sauce	30 mL
1 tbsp	cornstarch	15 mL
2 tsp	stevia brown sugar blend (such as Truvia or Splenda)	10 mL
2 tsp	unseasoned rice vinegar	10 mL
2 tsp	Thai chile sauce (such as Sriracha)	10 mL
1 tsp	garlic powder	5 mL
1	green bell pepper, cut into 1-inch (2.5 cm) strips	1
1	red bell pepper, cut into 1-inch (2.5 cm) strips	1
1 tsp	toasted sesame oil	5 mL

1. In a large sauté pan, heat 2 tsp (10 mL) of the olive oil over medium heat. When the oil is shimmering, add the tofu and cook on all sides, about 12 minutes. Remove the tofu to a clean plate.

2. Fill a medium saucepan with 1 inch (2.5 cm) of water and fit with a steamer basket. Add the green beans, cover and bring to a boil over high heat. Steam until the green beans are cooked but crisp, 3 to 5 minutes. Transfer to a clean bowl.

3. In a small bowl, whisk together the vegetable broth, soy sauce, cornstarch, brown sugar blend, rice vinegar, Thai chile sauce and garlic powder.

NUTRIENTS per serving	CALORIES 269.98	FAT 16.38 g	CARBOHYDRATE 17.83 g	PROTEIN 14.17 g	FIBER 5.12 g

4 In the pan used to cook the tofu, heat the remaining 2 tbsp (30 mL) olive oil over medium heat. When the oil is shimmering, add the red and green bell peppers and cook, tossing frequently, until slightly softened, about 8 minutes. Add the green beans and cooked tofu and toss to combine. Add the vegetable broth mixture and stir to evenly coat the vegetables. Reduce the heat to medium-low and simmer until the mixture thickens, 1 to 2 minutes. Add the toasted sesame oil and stir to combine.

5 **TO STORE:** In each of four containers, add 2 cups (500 mL) of the mixture. Cover and refrigerate for up to 4 days or freeze for up to 2 months.

6 **TO SERVE:** If frozen, thaw overnight in the refrigerator. To reheat, microwave uncovered on High for 90 seconds. Allow the heat to distribute for 2 minutes before removing the container from the microwave. Serve warm.

Tofu: A Healthy Protein

Tofu is a valuable source of plant-based protein, containing essential amino acids, iron and calcium. Tofu is a heart-healthy protein alternative to animal proteins.

Tips for Using Tofu

- Press tofu before cooking to remove excess water, allowing it to absorb marinades and sauces better.
- Marinate tofu in your favorite sauce or spices for added flavor before cooking.
- Tofu can be baked, grilled, sautéed or stir-fried.
- Use firm or extra-firm tofu for stir-fries and grilling, and silken tofu for smoothies, desserts and sauces.

Bok Choy, Tofu and Shiitake Stir-Fry

This classic combo of greens, meaty mushrooms and saucy tofu adds up to a vegetarian delight. Serve it over rice or Asian noodles.

Wok

TIPS

To prepare the bok choy for this recipe: Trim the base, then slice the head lengthwise into quarters. Slice each quarter crosswise into 1-inch (2.5 cm) pieces.

To maintain more control over the saltiness of dishes, use reduced-sodium soy sauce. Depending on the type, 1 tbsp (15 mL) regular soy sauce can contain 1,000 mg sodium or more. Reduced-sodium soy sauce contains about half that amount.

For the finest minced garlic, push it through a press.

To grate or purée gingerroot, use a kitchen rasp such as the type made by Microplane.

¼ cup	vegetable stock	60 mL
1 tbsp	soy sauce (see Tips)	15 mL
1 tsp	toasted sesame oil	5 mL
1 tsp	granulated sugar	5 mL
½ tsp	hot pepper flakes	2 mL
2 tbsp	oil, divided	30 mL
1	head bok choy (1¼ lbs/625 g), sliced into 1-inch (2.5 cm) pieces (see Tips)	1
1 tsp	kosher or coarse sea salt, divided	5 mL
4 oz	shiitake mushrooms, stemmed and thickly sliced	125 g
2	cloves garlic, minced (see Tips)	2
1 tsp	puréed gingerroot (see Tips)	5 mL
8 oz	medium-firm tofu, drained and cut into ½-inch (1 cm) cubes	250 g

1 In a small bowl, combine stock, soy sauce, sesame oil, sugar and hot pepper flakes. Set aside.

2 Heat a wok over medium-high heat for 1 minute. Swirl in 1 tbsp (15 mL) oil. Add bok choy and ½ tsp (2 mL) salt. Stir quickly to coat, then cook without disturbing for about 2 minutes, until tender-crisp. Transfer to a bowl and set aside.

3 Swirl remaining oil in wok. Add mushrooms and remaining salt. Stir-fry for 3 to 4 minutes, until they are softened, start to turn golden and sound squeaky. Push mushrooms to one side of wok. To center of wok, add garlic and ginger; stir-fry for 20 seconds. Add tofu and shake wok to combine. Add bok choy and prepared stock mixture. Stir-fry for about 1 minute, until sauce bubbles and thickens. Serve immediately.

NUTRIENTS	CALORIES	FAT	CARBOHYDRATE	PROTEIN	FIBER
per serving	154	11.5 g	6.8 g	9.2 g	2.3 g

Green Pad See Ew

MAKES 4 TO 6 SERVINGS

In this leafy green vegetarian version of a signature Thai dish, slippery rice noodles are bathed in a simple soy-lime sauce, while tofu and egg provide additional protein. Make sure you have all the ingredients prepped and ready, or what should be a simple job will become massively confusing.

Wok

TIPS

To prepare Chinese broccoli for this recipe: Trim, separating stems from leaves and florets. Using a vegetable peeler, peel the thickest stems and cut in half lengthwise. Cut stems crosswise into ½-inch (1 cm) pieces. Coarsely chop leaves and florets.

¼ cup	soy sauce	60 mL
1 tbsp	freshly squeezed lime juice	15 mL
1 tbsp	granulated sugar	15 mL
2	large eggs, optional	2
	Kosher or coarse sea salt	
8 oz	dried rice noodles, ½ inch (1 cm) wide	250 g
¼ cup	oil	60 mL
12 oz	medium tofu, drained and cut into ½-inch (1 cm) cubes	375 g
6	cloves garlic, slivered	6
1 lb	Chinese broccoli, stems, leaves and florets, separated and cut (see Tips)	500 g
2 tbsp	vegetable stock or water	30 mL
2 tbsp	slivered basil leaves	30 mL

1. In a small measuring cup, combine soy sauce, lime juice and sugar.

2. In a small bowl, lightly whisk eggs (if using) with salt to taste.

3. In a large pan of boiling salted water over medium heat, cook noodles for 5 to 8 minutes, until tender but firm. Drain.

4. Meanwhile, heat wok over high heat for 1 minute. Add oil and swirl to coat bottom of pan. Add eggs (if using) and fry undisturbed for about 1 minute, until very puffy. Flip over and then, using a slotted spoon, transfer to a large plate, leaving oil in wok. Using a spoon, break egg into large chunks.

5. In wok over high heat, add tofu (be careful, as it will spatter) and cook, shaking pan often, for 3 to 5 minutes, until golden. Using a slotted spoon, transfer tofu to a plate, leaving oil in wok.

6. Add garlic to wok and stir-fry for 20 seconds. Add Chinese broccoli, salt lightly to taste, and stir-fry for about 1 minute, until leaves are slightly wilted. Add stock, cover and cook for 3 to 4 minutes, until stems are tender-crisp. Add noodles and soy sauce mixture and, using tongs, toss gently to combine. Add eggs and toss briefly. Remove from heat. Season with salt to taste. Transfer to a serving platter or individual bowls. Top with tofu and sprinkle with basil. Serve immediately.

NUTRIENTS	CALORIES	FAT	CARBOHYDRATE	PROTEIN	FIBER
per serving	374	15.1 g	48 g	13.9 g	4 g

Whole Wheat Pasta with Spring Vegetables and Edamame

MAKES 6 SERVINGS

SERVING SIZE: 2 CUPS (500 ML) PASTA, 1 TBSP (15 ML) WALNUTS

This light and refreshing dish is perfect for a warm spring lunch or dinner. Use seasonal non-starchy vegetables that you have on hand to help reduce food waste in your kitchen.

TIP

If you prefer, swap the shelled edamame for lima beans.

¼ cup	raw walnuts, coarsely chopped	60 mL
10 oz	whole wheat rotini	300 g
1½ cups	shelled edamame	375 mL
	Zest and juice of 1 lemon	
¼ cup	grated Parmesan cheese	60 mL
¼ cup plus 1 tbsp	olive oil, divided	75 mL
2 tsp	dried parsley flakes	10 mL
½ tsp	salt	2 mL
¼ tsp	ground black pepper	1 mL
⅛ tsp	hot pepper flakes	0.5 mL
1	onion, chopped	1
2	cloves garlic, minced	2
1	zucchini, halved lengthwise and cut into ½-inch (1 cm) half-moons	1
2	carrots, peeled and shredded	2
1 cup	cherry tomatoes	250 mL

1 Heat a small skillet over medium-low heat. When the skillet is hot, add the walnuts and toast until fragrant, being careful not to burn the nuts, about 3 minutes. Transfer the toasted nuts to a clean bowl and set aside.

2 Fill a large pot three-quarters with water and bring to a boil over high heat. Add the rotini and reduce the heat to medium. Boil gently until the pasta is al dente, 10 minutes. Add the edamame to a colander and drain the pasta by pouring it over the edamame. Reserve about ½ cup (125 mL) of the pasta water.

3 In a small bowl, make the sauce by whisking together the lemon juice and zest, Parmesan cheese, ¼ cup (60 mL) of the olive oil, parsley, salt, black pepper and hot pepper flakes.

4 In a large saucepan, heat the remaining 1 tbsp (15 mL) olive oil over medium heat. When the oil is shimmering, add the onion and garlic and cook until the onion is translucent and the garlic is fragrant, 3 minutes. Add the bell pepper, zucchini and carrots and cook until the vegetables soften slightly, about 5 minutes.

NUTRIENTS per serving	CALORIES 371.93	FAT 16.63 g	CARBOHYDRATE 45.49 g	PROTEIN 12.67 g	FIBER 8.08 g

5   Add the tomatoes and toss for 1 minute more. Add the lemon sauce, pasta and edamame to the saucepan and toss to combine. If the pasta seems dry, add the reserved pasta water, a little bit at a time.

6   **TO STORE:** In each of four containers, add 2 cups (500 mL) of the pasta. Sprinkle each container with 1 tbsp (15 mL) of the toasted walnuts. Cover and refrigerate for up to 4 days or freeze for up to 2 months.

7   **TO SERVE:** If frozen, thaw in the refrigerator overnight. To reheat, microwave uncovered on High for 90 seconds. Allow 2 minutes for the heat to distribute before removing the container from the microwave. Serve warm.

Whole-Grain Pasta: A Fiber-Rich and Healthy Choice

Whole-grain pasta is rich in dietary fiber, vitamins and minerals, which aids digestion, promotes satiety, helps regulate blood sugar levels and maintain a healthy weight. The fiber in whole-grain pasta serves as a prebiotic, promoting the growth of beneficial gut bacteria that produce short-chain fatty acids that help decrease inflammation.

Tips for Cooking Whole-Grain Pasta

- Whole-grain pasta may require longer cooking times than refined pasta, so read the instructions.
- Pair the whole-grain pasta with vegetables, lean proteins and healthy fats.
- Add some tomato sauce and seasonings (basil, garlic) to enhance the flavor of whole-grain pasta.
- Store whole-grain pasta in a cool, dry place to maintain freshness.

Fettuccine with Fennel and Artichokes

Here is a spare-sauced pasta that is quick to make but as elegant as a more belabored creation. The only tricky bit is the final assembly and integration into the sauce, which must be handled carefully (it can be messy) and efficiently so that each portion gets its share of the treats. This recipe can be enriched by adding (at the last minute, in Step 3) cooked chicken strips, pancetta (Italian bacon), sautéed shrimp (or any other seafood), or sautéed mushrooms.

TIP

The fennel bulb always comes attached to woody branches and thin leaves that look like dill. You'll need the leaves for the final garnish, so cut them off and set them aside. Cut off and discard the woody branches. Quarter the bulb vertically, then cut out and discard the hard triangular sections of core. What remains is the usable part of the fennel.

¼ cup	olive oil	60 mL
½ tsp	salt	2 mL
¼ tsp	freshly ground black pepper	1 mL
½ tsp	fennel seeds	2 mL
1	fennel bulb, trimmed, cored and cut into ½-inch (1 cm) pieces (about 2 cups/500 mL)	1
1	medium tomato, cut into ½-inch (1 cm) wedges	1
4	sun-dried tomatoes, thinly sliced	4
1 tsp	balsamic vinegar	5 mL
1 tsp	dried basil	5 mL
1	jar (6 oz/170 mL) marinated artichoke hearts, drained	1
¼ cup	white wine	50 mL
1 lb	fettuccine	500 g
	Shredded sharp Italian cheese (such as pecorino, Crotonese, aged provolone or Romano)	
	Several sprigs fresh basil and/or parsley, chopped	

1 In a large deep frying pan, heat olive oil, salt, pepper and fennel seeds for 1 minute over high heat. Add fresh fennel pieces; sauté for 3 minutes or until the fennel is beginning to color. Add tomato wedges, sun-dried tomatoes, vinegar and dried basil; cook, stirring, for 2 to 3 minutes or until the tomato has broken down and a sauce is forming. Add artichokes and wine, reduce heat to medium and cook, stirring, for 2 minutes or until the sauce is bubbling again. Take off heat and reserve in frying pan.

2 In a large pot of boiling salted water, cook the fettuccine until tender but firm; drain.

3 Return frying pan to medium heat. Add the fettuccine. Toss and combine for 1 to 2 minutes or until all the pasta is coated with the sauce. Serve immediately, garnished with cheese and herbs.

NUTRIENTS per serving	CALORIES 706	FAT 19.4 g	CARBOHYDRATE 98.1 g	PROTEIN 21.8 g	FIBER 8.3 g

Penne with Eggplant and Mushrooms

This pasta dish has a messy, peasant look and feel to it, making it ideal for a casual get-together. The sweetness of the boiled-then-sautéed eggplant melts into the sauce, giving the dish its "informal" look, while providing a feast for the tastebuds. The assembly of sauce with pasta in Step 4 requires care and patience to ensure thorough integration.

2 cups	cubed peeled eggplant	500 mL
¼ cup	olive oil	60 mL
½ tsp	salt	2 mL
¼ tsp	freshly ground black pepper	1 mL
6 oz	wild or button mushrooms, trimmed and halved	175 g
4	cloves garlic, thinly sliced	4
1	medium tomato, cut into ½-inch (1 cm) wedges	1
1 tsp	dried basil	5 mL
½ tsp	balsamic vinegar	2 mL
¼ cup	water	60 mL
12 oz	penne noodles	375 g
	Few sprigs fresh basil and/or parsley, chopped	
	Grated Romano cheese	

1 Bring a pot of salted water to the boil while peeling and cutting eggplant. (Keep in mind that eggplant doesn't like to wait long after it's cut and will quickly turn brown.) Add eggplant to the boiling water, reduce heat to medium and cook 5 to 6 minutes or until eggplant is tender and softened. Drain and set aside.

2 In a large deep frying pan, heat olive oil, salt and pepper over high heat for 1 minute. Add mushrooms and eggplant; stir-fry for 3 minutes or until mushrooms are softened and eggplant begins to break up. Add garlic and stir-fry for 30 seconds. Add tomato, basil and vinegar; cook, stirring, for 2 to 3 minutes or until the tomato has broken down and a sauce is forming. Add water, reduce heat to medium and cook, stirring, for 1 minute or until the sauce is bubbling again. Take off heat and reserve in frying pan.

3 In a large pot of boiling salted water, cook the penne until tender but firm; drain.

4 Return frying pan to medium heat. Add the penne. Toss and combine for 1 to 2 minutes or until all the pasta is coated with the sauce. Serve immediately, garnished with cheese and herbs.

NUTRIENTS	CALORIES	FAT	CARBOHYDRATE	PROTEIN	FIBER
per serving	526	19.1 g	71.8 g	17.4 g	5 g

Mushroom-Spinach Lasagna with Goat Cheese

MAKES 4 TO 6 SERVINGS

Lasagna layered with meat, cheese and tomato sauce is so much a part of our gastronomic vocabulary that contemplating one with different ingredients requires a considerable stretch of the imagination. Still, there's a world of lasagnas out there. So if you're in the mood for a change, try this meatless variety—it's every bit as satisfying as the original.

Preheat oven to 375° F (190° C)

13- by 9-inch baking dish

TIPS

If expense or calories are a concern, you can substitute low-fat ricotta for the goat cheese in the filling, as well as 12 oz (375 g) low-fat mozzarella instead of the recommended mixture for the topping.

For noodles, either cook your own or use the "ready to bake" variety (preferably white ones, to contrast with the spinach).

12 oz	spinach, washed and trimmed	375 g
¼ cup	olive oil	50 mL
¾ tsp	salt	4 mL
½ tsp	freshly ground black pepper	2 mL
12 oz	portobello mushrooms, trimmed and sliced ½-inch (1 cm) thick	375 g
2 tbsp	finely chopped garlic	30 mL
½ tsp	chili flakes	2 mL
2 cups	finely diced peeled tomatoes, with juices, or canned tomatoes	500 mL
1 tsp	balsamic vinegar	5 mL
½ tsp	dried rosemary, crumbled	2 mL
½ tsp	dried thyme	2 mL
9	cooked lasagna noodles	9
8 oz	goat cheese	250 g
8 oz	shredded mozzarella (about 2 cups/500 mL)	250 g
4 oz	grated strong Italian cheese (such as Crotonese, Asiago or aged Provolone)	125 g

1. In a large pot, bring about 1 inch (2.5 cm) salted water to boil. Add spinach, cover and cook for 1 minute. Uncover, turn the spinach, cover again and cook 1 minute more. Drain. Rinse under cold water; drain. Press lightly to extract more water and set aside in a colander to continue draining.

2. In a large nonstick frying pan, heat 2 tbsp (30 mL) of the olive oil, ¼ tsp (0.5 mL) of the salt and ¼ tsp (0.5 mL) of the pepper over high heat for 1 minute. Add mushroom slices (they'll absorb all the oil immediately); stir-fry for 3 to 4 minutes or until browned and shiny. Add 1 tbsp (15 mL) of the garlic and stir-fry for 1 minute or until the garlic starts to brown. Transfer to a bowl and set aside.

3. In the same frying pan, heat remaining olive oil, remaining salt, remaining pepper, chili flakes and remaining garlic over high heat for 1 minute, stirring. Add tomatoes, vinegar, rosemary and thyme; cook, stirring, until bubbling. Cook, stirring, for 2 more minutes or until the tomatoes are breaking up and a sauce forms. Remove from heat and set aside.

NUTRIENTS	CALORIES	FAT	CARBOHYDRATE	PROTEIN	FIBER
per serving	652	37.9 g	45.1 g	35.2 g	5.7 g

4 Spread the bottom of baking dish with 2 tbsp (25 mL) of the tomato sauce. Lay flat 3 of the lasagna noodles (they should cover the whole surface). Spread the spinach evenly over the surface. Dot half of the goat cheese evenly over the spinach. Cover with another layer of 3 noodles. Spread the mushrooms evenly over lasagna noodles. Dot remaining goat cheese over the mushrooms. Cover with the last layer of 3 noodles and spoon the rest of the tomato sauce evenly over the noodles. Mix the grated mozzarella and strong Italian cheeses; sprinkle evenly over the surface of the lasagna to create the topping.

5 Bake uncovered for 35 to 40 minutes or until the topping is rosy-browned and the inside is bubbling. Remove from oven and let rest, uncovered, for 10 minutes to temper. Lift portions carefully to retain the cheese on top and serve immediately.

CHAPTER 8

Soups and Salads

Avgolemono   192

Roasted Carrot Soup with Pesto   193

Chicken and Wild Rice Soup   194

Ginger Pumpkin Soup   195

Higher Morels Creamy Mushroom Soup   196

Southwest Slaw   197

All Greens Salad with Lemon Vinaigrette   198

Lemon Vinaigrette   199

Crunchy Fennel Salad   200

Citrus Fennel Slaw   201

Three-Pea and Mint Salad   202

Tuscan White Bean and Tomato Salad   203

Chickpea and Roasted Red Pepper Salad   204

Grilled Corn and Lima Bean Salad   205

Black-Eyed Pea Salad with Tomato and Feta   206

Red Wine Vinaigrette   207

Garlic Herb Vinaigrette   208

Lemon Cumin Dressing   209

Homemade Mayonnaise   210

Classic Aïoli   211

More Dressings and Sauces

See the Lunch and Dinner chapters for these dressings and sauces:

Cucumber-Mango Raita   141

Sesame-Miso Garlic Dressing   147

Red Enchilada Sauce   167

Avgolemono

NUTRITION TIP
Replace the white rice with brown, red or wild rice for a more nutritious meal.

8 cups	chicken broth	2 L
¾ cup	long-grain white rice	175 mL
	Salt and freshly ground black pepper to taste	
3	egg yolks	3
	Juice of 2 lemons	
	Chopped chives	
	Additional chicken broth, chilled (if serving cold)	

In a large saucepan, bring broth to a boil.

Add rice, salt and pepper, reduce heat and simmer for 12 to 15 minutes, or until rice is tender.

Meanwhile, combine egg yolks and lemon juice. Slowly whisk 2 cups (500 mL) of the hot soup into egg mixture.

Reduce heat so that soup barely simmers and slowly pour in egg mixture, stirring constantly.

Increase heat to medium and cook, stirring, until soup thickens slightly (do not boil).

Serve hot or cold, garnished with chives.

If served cold, thin to desired consistency with chilled broth.

Variation

Lemon Chicken Soup with Orzo: Follow preceding recipe, but substitute orzo or another pastina for the rice.

Vitamin C

The lemons in this recipe provide gout-friendly vitamin C. Here is a list of fruits with high Vitamin C content. Remember that the actual amount can vary based on the size of the fruit and how ripe it is.
- **Guavas:** 228 mg per 100 grams
- **Blackcurrants:** 181 mg per 100 grams
- **Kiwi:** 93 mg per 100 grams
- **Strawberries:** 59 mg per 100 grams
- **Oranges:** 53 mg per 100 grams
- **Papayas:** 60 mg per 100 grams
- **Lemons:** 53 mg per 100 grams
- **Pineapple:** 48 mg per 100 grams

NUTRIENTS per serving	CALORIES	FAT	CARBOHYDRATE	PROTEIN	FIBER
	119	2.7 g	19.3 g	4.5 g	1 g

Roasted Carrot Soup with Pesto

MAKES 6 SERVINGS

SERVING SIZE: 1¼ CUPS (310 ML)

This warming soup is perfect on a cold, rainy day, but it's also a gorgeous option to serve for special occasions. The swirl of green pesto pops against the bright orange of the carrot, so it's the perfect starter for when you want to impress.

Preheat oven to 400°F (200°C)

2 rimmed baking sheets lined with parchment paper or a silicone mat

Blender

2 lbs	carrots, sliced into 1-inch (2.5 cm) rounds	1 kg
3 tbsp	olive oil, divided	45 mL
½ tsp	salt, divided	2 mL
¼ tsp	ground black pepper, divided	1 mL
1	onion, chopped	1
2	garlic cloves, crushed	2
3 cups	low-sodium vegetable broth	750 mL
3 cups	water	750 mL
½ tsp	ground coriander	2 mL
¼ tsp	ground cumin	1 mL
2 tbsp	prepared pesto	30 mL

1 In a large bowl, combine the carrots, 2 tbsp (30 mL) olive oil, ¼ tsp (1 mL) salt and ⅛ tsp (0.5 mL) pepper. Spread the carrots in a single layer on the prepared baking sheets. Roast in the preheated oven, turning halfway through, until the carrots are slightly browned and fragrant, about 25 minutes. Remove from the oven and let cool for 5 minutes.

2 Meanwhile, in a large saucepan, heat the remaining 1 tbsp (15 mL) olive oil over medium heat until shimmering. Add the onion and garlic; cook, stirring occasionally, until the onion is translucent, about 3 minutes. Add the roasted carrots, vegetable broth, water, coriander, cumin and the remaining ¼ tsp (1 mL) salt and ⅛ tsp (0.5 mL) pepper; raise the heat to high and bring to a boil. Reduce the heat to medium-low, cover and simmer, stirring occasionally, until the flavors meld, about 20 minutes. Set aside to cool slightly, about 15 to 20 minutes.

3 In a blender, working in batches as necessary, blend the cooled carrot mixture on high speed until smooth, about 1 minute.

4 Ladle 1¼ cups (310 mL) soup into each of 6 bowls. Dollop 1 tsp (5 mL) pesto in each bowl and swirl it into the soup.

NUTRIENTS	CALORIES	FAT	CARBOHYDRATE	PROTEIN	FIBER
per serving	189	12 g	20 g	3 g	6 g

Chicken and Wild Rice Soup

Not only does wild rice soup taste fantastic, it seems to have the magical power to warm you to your bones.

Instant Pot

2 tbsp	butter	30 mL
1 cup	chopped onion	250 mL
1 cup	diced carrots	250 mL
1 cup	diced celery	250 mL
2	boneless skinless chicken breasts, cut into cubes	2
1	package (6 oz/175 g) long-grain and wild rice mix	1
1 tbsp	dried parsley	15 mL
1 tsp	kosher salt	5 mL
½ tsp	freshly ground black pepper	2 mL
1¾ cups	ready-to-use chicken broth	425 mL
1 tbsp	cornstarch	15 mL
2 tbsp	cold water	30 mL
4 oz	brick-style cream cheese, cubed	125 g
1 cup	milk	250 mL
1 cup	half-and-half (10%) cream	250 mL

1 Press Sauté on the Instant Pot; the indicator will read "Normal." When the display says "Hot," add butter to the pot and heat until melted. Add onion, carrots and celery; cook, stirring, for 4 to 5 minutes or until tender. Press Cancel. Add chicken, rice mix (without any seasoning packet), parsley, salt, pepper and broth, stirring well.

2 Close and lock the lid and turn the steam release handle to Sealing. Press Manual; the indicator will read "High Pressure." Use the ⊖ button to decrease the time on the display to 7 minutes.

3 When the timer beeps, press Cancel and let the pot stand, covered, for 5 minutes. After 5 minutes, turn the steam release handle to Venting and remove the lid. Check to make sure the chicken is no longer pink inside. (If more cooking is needed, reset the manual pressure to "High Pressure" for 1 minute.)

4 In a small bowl, whisk together cornstarch and cold water. Press Sauté. Stir the cornstarch mixture into the pot. Add cream cheese and stir until melted. Add milk and cream; cook, stirring, until heated through (do not let boil).

Variation

For a vegetarian version, use vegetable broth and omit the chicken.

NUTRIENTS	CALORIES	FAT	CARBOHYDRATE	PROTEIN	FIBER
per serving	379	17.7 g	34.7 g	19.7 g	2.2 g

Ginger Pumpkin Soup

MAKES 6 SERVINGS

This colorful soup has so many things going for it, you just must give it a try. It boasts a combination of sweet, spicy, zesty and creamy flavors and is perfect as a main dish or as a starter for an Indian-inspired meal.

Instant Pot

TIPS

Use pie pumpkins (also known as sugar pumpkins or sweet pumpkins), as they are much more flavorful than the larger ones typically used for decorating or carving.

This soup can be completed through Step 3 and then refrigerated in airtight containers for up to 1 week.

To chiffonade basil, remove the stems and stack 10 or more leaves. Roll the leaves up lengthwise into a fairly tight spiral, then cut crosswise into thin strips. Fluff the strips.

3 tbsp	butter	45 mL
3	cloves garlic, minced	3
1	large onion, minced	1
2 tbsp	minced gingerroot	30 mL
1 tsp	ground cumin	5 mL
½ tsp	curry powder	2 mL
4 cups	cubed seeded peeled pie pumpkin	1 L
2 tbsp	packed brown sugar	30 mL
1 tbsp	kosher salt	15 mL
3½ cups	water	875 mL
1⅔ cups	coconut milk	400 mL
2 tsp	sweet Thai chile sauce (optional)	10 mL
	Juice of 1 orange	
1 cup	plain Greek yogurt	250 mL
	Grated zest of 1 lime	
¼ cup	fresh basil chiffonade (see Tip)	60 mL

1. Press Sauté on the Instant Pot; the indicator will read "Normal." When the display says "Hot," add butter to the pot and heat until melted. Add garlic, onion, ginger, cumin and curry powder; cook, stirring, for 4 to 5 minutes or until onion is soft and spices are fragrant. Press Cancel. Add pumpkin, brown sugar, salt, water, coconut milk, chile sauce (if using) and orange juice, stirring well.

2. Close and lock the lid and turn the steam release handle to Sealing. Press Manual; the indicator will read "High Pressure." Press Pressure once to adjust the pressure to "Low Pressure." Use the ⊖ button to decrease the time on the display to 3 minutes.

3. When the timer beeps, press Cancel and turn the steam release handle to Venting. When the float valve drops down, remove the lid. The pumpkin should be very tender when tested with a fork. (If more cooking is needed, reset the manual pressure to "Low Pressure" for 1 minute.) Stir soup well and adjust seasoning, if desired.

4. In a small bowl, combine yogurt and lime zest. Ladle soup into serving bowls and serve dolloped with lime yogurt and garnished with basil.

NUTRIENTS	CALORIES	FAT	CARBOHYDRATE	PROTEIN	FIBER
per serving	267	20 g	20.9 g	5 g	3.1 g

Higher Morels Creamy Mushroom Soup

MAKES 4 SERVINGS

Blender

¼ cup	olive oil	60 mL
2 lbs	cremini mushrooms, chopped	1 kg
1	small onion, chopped	1
	Sea salt	
4	garlic cloves, minced	4
⅓ cup	unbleached all-purpose flour	75 mL
	Water	
3	cubes (each 1 tsp/5 mL) no-beef or vegetable bouillon	3
1	bay leaf	1
1 tsp	dried thyme	5 mL
	Freshly ground black pepper	

1. In a large pot, heat olive oil over medium-high heat. Add mushrooms, onion and ½ tsp (2 mL) sea salt; cook, stirring occasionally, for 3 to 5 minutes, until mushrooms have released their liquid. Reduce heat to medium and add garlic; cook, stirring often, for about 15 minutes, until mushrooms are swimming in their own liquid.

2. Add flour and toss to coat mushrooms. Cook, stirring constantly, for 3 minutes, or until flour turns dark beige. Do not allow the flour to brown. If it becomes too dry, add 1 tbsp (15 mL) water at a time, until a paste forms.

3. Stir in bouillon, bay leaf, thyme and 8 cups (2 L) water; bring to a boil over high heat. Reduce heat to medium-low, partially cover, and simmer for 15 to 20 minutes, until thickened slightly.

4. Remove bay leaf and let soup cool slightly. Working in batches as necessary, transfer soup to the blender. Remove the plug in the lid and blend on high speed until smooth.

5. Return the blended soup to the pot and give it a good stir. Heat over medium until warmed.

6. Season to taste with sea salt and pepper; serve.

Hack It
Make this recipe gluten-free by substituting cornstarch for the flour.

NUTRIENTS	CALORIES	FAT	CARBOHYDRATE	PROTEIN	FIBER
per serving	236	14.8 g	21 g	9.2 g	3.5 g

Southwest Slaw

MAKES 6 SERVINGS

Northern winters are long and chilly, and the variety of available fresh vegetables shrinks dramatically. That's when we have to get creative with cabbage and carrots and such. This tasty creamy slaw is popular all year long.

Food processor with slicing blade or mandolin, optional

¼	head red cabbage	¼
¼	head green cabbage	¼
1	carrot	1
1	red bell pepper	1
1	jalapeño pepper, seeded	1
¾ cup	mayonnaise	175 mL
1 tbsp	Dijon mustard	15 mL
1 tbsp	natural rice vinegar	15 mL
2 tsp	freshly squeezed lime juice	10 mL
2 tsp	brown sugar	10 mL
1 tsp	minced garlic	5 mL
1 tsp	toasted cumin seeds	5 mL
	Kosher or sea salt	
2 tbsp	chopped cilantro	30 mL

1 Cut out and discard hard core of red and green cabbages. Cut cabbages into fine slivers or shred in a food processor with a slicing blade or using a mandolin. Transfer to a large bowl and set aside.

2 Slice carrot and bell and jalapeño peppers into juliennes. Add to cabbage.

3 In a small bowl, combine mayonnaise, mustard, vinegar, lime juice, brown sugar, garlic and cumin. Add dressing to vegetables and mix thoroughly. Season with salt to taste. Garnish with cilantro.

NUTRIENTS per serving	CALORIES 229	FAT 20.9 g	CARBOHYDRATE 9.7 g	PROTEIN 1.8 g	FIBER 2.8 g

All Greens Salad with Lemon Vinaigrette

MAKES 4 SERVINGS

SERVING SIZE: 2¾ CUPS (675 ML)

This dynamic salad is the perfect tasty way to get in your greens! For more protein, serve it alongside a piece of cooked fish, chicken or beef, or top with sautéed diced tofu or a hard-cooked egg.

TIP

If your asparagus spears are quite thin, the cooking time may be shortened by a few minutes.

8 oz	asparagus, trimmed and halved (see Tip)	250 g
½ cup	frozen peas	125 mL
6 cups	chopped romaine lettuce	1.5 L
2 tbsp	chopped fresh dill	30 mL
½	English cucumber, cut lengthwise and sliced into ½-inch (1 cm) half-moons	½
1	green bell pepper, cut into 1-inch (2.5 cm) strips	1
1	avocado, thinly sliced	1
½ cup	Lemon Vinaigrette (page 199)	125 mL

1. Add 1 inch (2.5 cm) water to a medium saucepan fitted with a steamer basket. Place the asparagus in the basket and bring the water to a boil over high heat. Reduce the heat to low, cover and steam until the asparagus is just tender, about 8 minutes. Using tongs, remove the asparagus from the steamer basket and transfer to a medium bowl.

2. Remove the steamer basket from the saucepan. Add water as necessary to maintain 1 inch (2.5 cm) in the pan; bring to a boil over high heat. Add the peas and cook until tender, about 5 minutes. Drain and add to the bowl with the asparagus.

3. In a large serving bowl, combine the lettuce and dill. Add the cucumber, bell pepper, cooked asparagus and peas. Just before serving, top with the avocado and add the Lemon Vinaigrette; toss to coat.

NUTRIENTS	CALORIES	FAT	CARBOHYDRATE	PROTEIN	FIBER
per serving	292	26 g	15 g	5 g	8 g

Lemon Vinaigrette

**MAKES 6 SERVINGS
(¾ CUP/175 ML)**

**SERVING SIZE: 2 TBSP
(30 ML)**

**This refreshing
vinaigrette
complements
pretty much
any green salad.**

¼ cup	apple cider vinegar	60 mL
Zest and juice of 1 lemon		
2 tsp	Dijon mustard	10 mL
1	garlic clove, minced	1
1 tsp	dried oregano	5 mL
1 tsp	dried parsley	5 mL
¼ tsp	salt	1 mL
⅛ tsp	ground black pepper	0.5 mL
½ cup	extra-virgin olive oil	125 mL

1. In a medium bowl, whisk together the apple cider vinegar, lemon zest, lemon juice, mustard, garlic, oregano, parsley, salt and pepper. Slowly drizzle in the olive oil, whisking constantly until incorporated.

2. Use immediately or cover and refrigerate for up to 2 weeks.

NUTRIENTS per serving	CALORIES 165	FAT 19 g	CARBOHYDRATE 1 g	PROTEIN 0 g	FIBER 0 g

Crunchy Fennel Salad

**SERVING SIZE: 1 CUP
(250 ML)**

Fennel tastes like anise, which may remind you of black licorice. It pairs beautifully with something sweet, such as mandarin oranges or apples (as in this recipe). I prefer to use sweeter apples here to balance the fennel flavor.

TIP

Swap the apple for a medium red Anjou pear.

2 tbsp	apple cider vinegar	30 mL
1 tsp	liquid honey	5 mL
¼ tsp	salt	1 mL
¼ cup	extra-virgin olive oil	60 mL
1	medium bulb fennel, trimmed, quartered and thinly sliced	1
6	medium radishes, halved and thinly sliced	1
1	medium apple, such as Honeycrisp, Gala or Fuji, quartered and thinly sliced	1
½ cup	roughly chopped walnuts	125 mL
2 tbsp	shredded Romano cheese	30 mL

1 In a small bowl, whisk together the apple cider vinegar, honey and salt. Slowly drizzle in the olive oil, whisking constantly until incorporated.

2 In a large bowl, combine the fennel, radishes and apple. Just before serving, add the vinegar mixture and toss to coat. Top with the walnuts and Romano cheese. Serve immediately.

NUTRIENTS	CALORIES	FAT	CARBOHYDRATE	PROTEIN	FIBER
per serving	134	11 g	8 g	2 g	2 g

Citrus Fennel Slaw

MAKES 6 SERVINGS

The fennel and citrus combination is a natural in this crunchy twist on coleslaw. Kids enjoy the citrus flavors.

TIPS

To get thin, even slices, use a mandoline to cut the fennel bulb.

Instead of serving on top of greens on individual plates, you can also simply pass the slaw.

Jaclyn Pritchard, Dietitian, Ontario

1	large fennel bulb	1
¼	red onion, very thinly sliced	¼
	Grated zest and juice of 1 lemon	
	Grated zest of 1 orange	
2 tbsp	freshly squeezed orange juice	30 mL
1 tbsp	canola oil	15 mL
Pinch	salt	Pinch
	Freshly ground black pepper	
6 cups	mesclun mix	1.5 L
3 tbsp	toasted pine nuts	45 mL

1. Remove the stalks and tough outer leaves of the fennel bulb and discard. Cut bulb in half lengthwise and trim out core. Cut bulb crosswise into very thin slices.

2. Place fennel slices and red onion in a large bowl. Stir in lemon zest, lemon juice, orange zest and orange juice. Drizzle with oil and sprinkle with salt and pepper to taste.

3. Divide mesclun mix evenly among six small plates. Mound one-sixth of the fennel slaw on each plate and garnish with pine nuts.

Variation

Substitute toasted unsalted sunflower seeds for the pine nuts.

NUTRIENTS per serving	CALORIES 85	FAT 5.4 g	CARBOHYDRATE 9 g	PROTEIN 2 g	FIBER 3 g

Three-Pea and Mint Salad

MAKES 6 SERVINGS

Here's a vibrant salad to welcome spring. Combine peas with dressing shortly before serving, since the bright color fades within a few hours.

TIP

To string edible-pod peas: With a sharp paring knife, cut across the stem end of the peas toward the inside edge and pull away the thin cellulose string that holds the two sides of the pod together.

3 cups	peas, fresh or frozen	750 mL
2 cups	snow peas (see Tip)	500 mL
1 cup	sugar snap peas	250 mL
1 tbsp	finely chopped shallot	15 mL
1 tbsp	mint chiffonade	15 mL
½ cup	White Wine Vinaigrette, omitting garlic (see Variation, page 207)	125 mL
	Kosher or sea salt	

1 Bring a large pot of lightly salted water to a boil. Add peas and cook until tender, 5 to 15 minutes. (Timing will vary depending on whether you are using fresh or frozen peas.) String snow peas and snap peas and blanch briefly, for 30 seconds. Drain and rinse under cold water to stop the cooking. Set aside.

2 In a large bowl, combine peas, shallot and mint. Toss with vinaigrette. Season with salt to taste.

NUTRIENTS	CALORIES	FAT	CARBOHYDRATE	PROTEIN	FIBER
per serving	187	13.9 g	11.9 g	4.5 g	3.9 g

Tuscan White Bean and Tomato Salad

MAKES 6 SERVINGS

A simple excellent salad that is very quick to prepare when using good quality canned white beans. We like to add variety and texture by making this salad with different varieties of dried beans or fava beans cooked in the kitchen.

TIP

For speed and convenience, replace dried beans with 1 can (14 to 19 oz/398 to 540 mL) white beans, rinsed and drained.

1 cup	dried white navy beans (see Tip)	250 mL
	Kosher or sea salt	
¼ cup	olive oil	60 mL
2 tsp	finely chopped garlic	10 mL
	Freshly ground black pepper	
2 cups	diced seeded ripe tomatoes	500 mL
¼	red onion, diced	¼
1 tbsp	coarsely chopped oregano	15 mL
2 tbsp	balsamic vinegar	30 mL

1. Place beans in a bowl and add water to cover. Set aside to soak overnight in the refrigerator. Drain beans.

2. In a saucepan over medium heat, add beans and cover with cold water, about 4 cups (1 L). Bring to a boil and cook until soft, 40 to 45 minutes. Remove from heat. Add a pinch of salt and let stand for 5 minutes. Drain and set aside.

3. In a large skillet, heat oil over medium-low heat. Add garlic and sauté until soft and just beginning to caramelize, 1 to 2 minutes. Add beans and toss to combine with garlic-infused oil. Season lightly with salt and pepper. Let cool.

4. In a large bowl, combine cooled beans, tomatoes, red onion, oregano and vinegar. Toss to combine well. Season with black pepper to taste.

NUTRIENTS	CALORIES	FAT	CARBOHYDRATE	PROTEIN	FIBER
per serving	216	9.5 g	25.5 g	8.8 g	7.1 g

Chickpea and Roasted Pepper Salad

MAKES 4 SERVINGS

This salad is quick and easy to prepare, tastes good and travels well. It's a perfect stand-by for summer picnics.

TIP

All canned chickpeas and beans are not created equal. In our kitchen we periodically taste-test different brands of canned goods. We advise you to do the same. We are always amazed at the different qualities of taste and texture. Even the same brand will differ from year to year. In this case we find a quality brand of organic legumes is superior. Remember to rinse off the preserving liquid and drain well before using.

1	roasted red bell pepper, diced	1
1	carrot, grated	1
2	cans (each 14 to 19 oz/398 to 540 mL) chickpeas, rinsed and drained (see Tip)	2
½ cup	Red Wine Vinaigrette (page 207)	125 mL
2 tbsp	chopped flat-leaf parsley	30 mL
2 tsp	chopped oregano	10 mL
	Salt and freshly ground black pepper	

1. In a large bowl, combine roasted pepper, carrot and chickpeas.
2. Add vinaigrette, parsley and oregano and toss to combine. Season with salt and pepper to taste.

Love Your Legumes

The Mediterranean diet recommends at least three servings of legumes per week. Here is a list of the most commonly used legumes and their protein content:

- **Lentils:** 1 cup (250 mL) cooked = 18 grams of protein
- **Chickpeas (garbanzo beans):** 1 cup (250 mL) cooked = 15 grams of protein
- **Black beans:** 1 cup (250 mL) cooked = 15 grams of protein
- **Soybeans:** 1 cup (250 mL) cooked = 29 grams of protein
- **Kidney beans:** 1 cup (250 mL) cooked = 15 grams of protein
- **Green peas:** 1 cup (250 mL) cooked = 9 grams of protein
- **Peanuts:** ¼ cup (60 mL) roasted = 9 grams of protein)

NUTRIENTS per serving	CALORIES	FAT	CARBOHYDRATE	PROTEIN	FIBER
	385	24.2 g	34 g	10.2 g	9.9 g

Grilled Corn and Lima Bean Salad

MAKES 4 TO 6 SERVINGS

This colorful, refreshing salad makes a satisfying lunch all by itself.

Preheated barbecue or indoor grill

TIP
Slicing kernels from a cob of corn: Make a slice across the bottom of the corncob so that it stands upright on a large cutting board. Hold the blade of a sharp knife against the cob at the top and slice downward firmly following the shape of the cob and releasing the kernels as you go.

2	ears corn, husk and silk removed (see Tip)	2
3 tbsp	olive oil, divided	45 mL
	Kosher or sea salt	
2 cups	frozen lima beans	500 mL
1 cup	halved cherry tomatoes	250 mL
1	shallot, diced	1
¼ cup	kalamata olives, pitted and roughly chopped	60 mL
2 tbsp	apple cider vinegar	30 mL
	Freshly ground black pepper	
1 cup	baby arugula	250 mL
½ cup	crumbled feta cheese	125 mL

1 Brush corn lightly with 1 tbsp (15 mL) of the oil and sprinkle with salt. Place on a lightly oiled grill over medium-high heat and grill until lightly charred on all sides. Let cool and slice kernels from the cob. Transfer to a large bowl and set aside.

2 In a saucepan of boiling lightly salted water, blanch lima beans until tender, 3 to 5 minutes. Drain and let cool. Add to corn with tomatoes, shallot and olives.

3 In a small bowl, whisk vinegar with remaining oil and season with salt and pepper to taste.

4 Pour dressing over vegetables and mix together well. Taste and adjust seasoning. Gently fold in arugula and feta.

NUTRIENTS	CALORIES	FAT	CARBOHYDRATE	PROTEIN	FIBER
per serving	470	11.5 g	73.3 g	21.2 g	16.7 g

Black-Eyed Pea Salad with Tomato and Feta

Double up the ingredients in this colorful salad and take along to a summer potluck. If the salad has to travel, combine black-eyed peas, onion and olives with the dressing and pack tomato, herbs and feta in small containers to add before serving.

TIP

For speed and convenience, replace dried beans with 1 can (14 to 19 oz/398 to 540 mL) black-eyed peas, rinsed and drained.

1 cup	dried black-eyed peas (see Tip)	250 mL
	Kosher or sea salt	
1	large ripe tomato, seeded and diced	1
½	red onion, chopped	½
¼ cup	kalamata olives, pitted and halved	60 mL
¼ cup	Red Wine Vinaigrette (page 207)	60 mL
2 tbsp	coarsely chopped flat-leaf parsley	30 mL
1 tbsp	finely chopped oregano	15 mL
½ cup	crumbled feta cheese	125 mL
	Freshly ground black pepper	

1. Place black-eyed peas in a bowl and add water to cover. Set aside to soak overnight in the refrigerator. Drain peas.

2. In a saucepan over medium heat, add black-eyed peas and cover with cold water, about 4 cups (1 L). Bring to a boil and cook until soft, 35 to 45 minutes. Remove from heat. Add a pinch of salt and let stand for 5 minutes. Drain. Transfer to a large bowl. Let cool.

3. Add tomato, red onion and olives. Add vinaigrette, parsley and oregano and toss to mix well. Season with salt to taste. Garnish with feta and a few grindings of black pepper.

NUTRIENTS	CALORIES	FAT	CARBOHYDRATE	PROTEIN	FIBER
per serving	248	12.8 g	24.1 g	10.7 g	4.8 g

Red Wine Vinaigrette

TIP
Read the ingredient label on most commercial salad dressings and you will see sugar fairly high on the list. Our collective taste buds obviously favor sweetness. If you find your homemade dressing too acidic to your taste, add a pinch of sugar or drizzle of honey.

We most frequently use the proportion of three parts oil to one part acidic ingredient (vinegar or citrus juice or a combination) in our salad dressings. However, the proportion may be adjusted to taste and will vary according to the individual characteristics of the oil and vinegar being used and the salad ingredients (e.g., bean salads benefit from a splash more acidity).

1 tsp	finely chopped garlic, optional	5 mL
1 tsp	Dijon mustard	5 mL
¼ tsp	kosher or sea salt	1 mL
2 tbsp	red wine vinegar	30 mL
6 tbsp	extra-virgin olive oil	90 mL
Pinch	freshly ground black pepper	Pinch
1 tbsp	freshly squeezed lemon juice, optional	15 m

1. In a small bowl, mash together garlic, if using, mustard and salt. Add vinegar. Slowly whisk in oil. Season with pepper to taste. Add lemon juice for a little fruity acidity, if needed.

Variation
White Wine Vinaigrette: Substitute white wine vinegar for red wine vinegar and proceed as above.

NUTRIENTS per serving	CALORIES 181	FAT 20.3 g	CARBOHYDRATE 0.1 g	PROTEIN 0.1 g	FIBER 0.1 g

Garlic Herb Vinaigrette

MAKES ⅓ CUP (75 ML)

**SERVING SIZE:
2 TBSP (30 ML)**

This is a perfectly balanced and versatile French vinaigrette. My master recipe includes parsley but I often switch to other herbs, depending on the salad ingredients and my mood.

TIP
For the finest minced garlic, push it through a press.

2 tbsp	white wine vinegar, divided	30 mL
1	clove garlic, minced (see Tip)	1
1 tbsp	finely chopped fresh parsley	15 mL
½ tsp	Dijon mustard	2 mL
½ tsp	granulated sugar 2 mL	
¼ tsp	kosher or coarse sea salt	1 mL
⅛ tsp	freshly ground black pepper	0.5 mL
¼ cup	extra-virgin olive oil	60 mL

1 In a bowl, whisk together 1½ tbsp (22 mL) vinegar, garlic, parsley, mustard, sugar, salt and pepper. Gradually whisk in oil. Add some or all of the remaining vinegar, if desired. Transfer to an airtight container and refrigerate for up to 1 week.

Variation
Garlic Basil Vinaigrette: Substitute an equal amount of basil for the parsley.

NUTRIENTS	CALORIES	FAT	CARBOHYDRATE	PROTEIN	FIBER
per serving	166	18 g	1.2 g	0.1 g	0.1 g

Lemon Cumin Dressing

**SERVING SIZE:
2 TBSP (30 ML)**

**A whiff of this and
my thoughts turn
to the compelling
cuisines of the
Mediterranean and
the Middle East.**

TIP
You can substitute black
pepper for the white
pepper. White pepper is
used mainly for aesthetic
reasons, to avoid black
specks in finished dishes.

2 tbsp	freshly squeezed lemon juice	30 mL
1	clove garlic, minced	1
2 tsp	liquid honey or vegan alternative	10 mL
1 tsp	kosher or coarse sea salt	5 mL
1 tsp	ground cumin	5 mL
1/8 tsp	freshly ground white pepper (see Tip)	0.5 mL
1/4 cup	extra-virgin olive oil	60 mL

1 In a bowl, whisk together lemon juice, garlic, honey, salt, cumin and pepper. Gradually whisk in oil. Transfer to an airtight container and refrigerate for up to 2 weeks.

NUTRIENTS per serving	CALORIES	FAT	CARBOHYDRATE	PROTEIN	FIBER
	180	18.2 g	5.2 g	0.2 g	0.2 g

Homemade Mayonnaise

**MAKES ABOUT 2 CUPS
(500 ML)**

**SERVING SIZE: 2 TBSP
(30 ML)**

TIP
If you are concerned
about the food safety of
raw eggs, you may wish
to skip this recipe.

Pinch	cayenne pepper	Pinch
	Salt and freshly ground white pepper to taste	
1 tbsp	boiling water	15 mL
2	large or extra-large egg yolks	2
2 tsp	Dijon mustard	10 mL
2 tbsp	freshly squeezed lemon juice	30 mL
1½ cups	bland vegetable oil (such as safflower, peanut, sunflower)	375 mL

1. In a bowl (or food processor), dissolve cayenne, salt and white pepper in boiling water.

2. Add egg yolks and mustard; beat with a whisk (or process) until lightly thickened.

3. Stir in lemon juice.

4. Add oil in a slow, steady stream (with the motor running, through the feed tube, if using a food processor), mixing constantly, until thick and creamy.

5. Adjust seasoning, if necessary.

NUTRIENTS	CALORIES	FAT	CARBOHYDRATE	PROTEIN	FIBER
per serving	188	21 g	0.2 g	0.4 g	0 g

Classic Aïoli

**MAKES ABOUT 1 CUP
(250 ML)**

**SERVING SIZE: 2 TBSP
(30 ML)**

**Aïoli is a garlic
mayonnaise that
goes well with all
types of seafood and
vegetables.**

Food processor

TIP

This recipe contains raw
egg yolks. If you are
concerned about the
safety of using raw eggs,
use pasteurized eggs
in the shell or ¼ cup
(60 mL) pasteurized
liquid whole eggs.

2	egg yolks (see Tip)	2
1½ cups	extra-virgin olive oil, divided	375 mL
1	clove garlic, coarsely chopped	1
1 tbsp	freshly squeezed lemon juice	15 mL
1 tsp	Dijon mustard	5 mL
¼ tsp	kosher salt	1 mL
¼ tsp	freshly ground black pepper	1 mL

1 In a food processor, process egg yolks for 2 minutes. With processor running, slowly drizzle ½ cup (125 mL) of the olive oil through the feed tube, until slightly thickened. (This must be done very slowly or the oil will not emulsify and your sauce will not thicken.) While processor is still running, add garlic, lemon juice and mustard and blend well.

2 Slowly add remaining olive oil until creamy and slightly thick. If too thick, turn processor back on and add 1 to 4 tsp (5 to 20 mL) water. Season with salt and pepper. Cover and refrigerate for 30 minutes. Store in refrigerator for up to 3 days.

NUTRIENTS	CALORIES	FAT	CARBOHYDRATE	PROTEIN	FIBER
per serving	373	41.6 g	0.5 g	0.8 g	0.1 g

CHAPTER 9

Sides

Roasted Lemon Asparagus   214

Sea Salt and Chile Shanghai Bok Choy   215

Sheet Pan Broccoli and Cauliflower   216

Brussels Sprouts with Almond Thyme Butter   217

Stir-Fried Brussels Sprouts   218

Sautéed Red Chard with Lemon and Pine Nuts   219

Eggplant with Tomatoes and Cumin   220

Garlicky Okra   221

Garlic Sautéed Spinach   222

Winter Greens with Split Yellow Peas / Saag aur Channa Dal   223

Sautéed Zucchini with Lemon and Pine Nuts   224

Ginger and Orange Braised Carrots   225

Honey Roasted Carrots   226

Oven-Roasted Mixed Veggies   227

Oven-Baked Sweet Potato Fries with Curry Mayo   228

Roasted Sweet Potatoes   229

Buttery Garlic Mashed Potatoes   230

Crushed Potatoes with Black Sesame Seeds/Kalay Tilawalle Aloo   231

Red Potatoes with Chives   232

Israeli Couscous and Mushrooms   233

Brown Rice with Peas and Carrots   234

Cayenne-Spiked Apricot and Nuts Pulao   235

Simple Rice Pilaf   236

Quinoa Pilaf   237

Tabbouleh with Lentils   238

Roasted Lemon Asparagus

This was the first dish Honey prepared in her own kitchen after getting married. It has loads of tang from the fresh lemon juice and zest, so pucker up!

Preheat oven to 350°F (180°C)

Rimmed baking sheet, lined with foil

TIPS

The baking time will vary depending on the width of the asparagus spears. Check occasionally for doneness.

For an extra flourish, sprinkle the cooked asparagus with 2 tbsp (30 mL) freshly grated Parmesan cheese.

You can also grill the asparagus, either on the baking sheet or in a grill basket on a barbecue grill preheated to medium-high.

Honey Bloomberg,
Dietitian, Ontario

1	bunch asparagus (about 1 lb/500 g), ends trimmed	1
1	lemon	1
2	cloves garlic, minced	2
2 tbsp	olive oil	30 mL
¼ tsp	salt	1 mL
¼ tsp	freshly ground black pepper	1 mL

1 Spread asparagus on prepared baking sheet. Grate zest and squeeze juice from ½ lemon into a small bowl. Stir in garlic, oil, salt and pepper. Pour over asparagus and shake pan to ensure each spear is coated.

2 Cut the remaining lemon half into slices and place among asparagus spears.

3 Bake in preheated oven, turning once, for 10 to 12 minutes or until lightly browned and tender-crisp.

Asparagus

References to asparagus go as far back as Egyptian hieroglyphics. There are many varieties, including wild, purple, variegated, green and white asparagus. White asparagus is grown under mounds of soil, so the plant gets no sunlight, blocking its ability to produce chlorophyll. Cook asparagus soon after you purchase it or the natural sugars will quickly turn to starch and the texture will be woody.

NUTRIENTS	CALORIES	FAT	CARBOHYDRATE	PROTEIN	FIBER
per serving	83	6.9 g	5 g	2 g	2 g

Sea Salt and Chile Shanghai Bok Choy

MAKES 4 SERVINGS

When you are short on time but long for flavor, this superfast and simple stir-fry hits the spot. Serve the crunchy bok choy over rice to capture its tasty juices.

Wok

TIPS

For the finest minced garlic, push it through a press.

Finger chiles are also known as cayenne peppers. They are slender, with pointed tips. You can substitute any kind of red chile you prefer.

Sea salt is light and flaky, and different types vary in saltiness. Adjust the amount according to your taste.

I use Shanghai bok choy in this recipe because it doesn't release as much water as white bok choy. To evaporate as much excess liquid as possible, cook this bok choy over high heat.

To sliver green onions, use a sharp knife to cut thin slices on an extreme diagonal from the root end to the stalk.

2	large cloves garlic, minced (see Tips)	2
1	large red finger chile, seeded and chopped (see Tips)	1
2 tsp	coarse sea salt (see Tips)	10 mL
1 tsp	granulated sugar 5 mL	
2 tbsp	oil	30 mL
2	large Shanghai bok choy (1 lb/500 g total), trimmed, halved lengthwise and cut crosswise into 1-inch (2.5 cm) pieces	2
2	green onions (white and green parts), slivered (see Tips)	2

1 In a small bowl, combine garlic, chile, salt and sugar. Set aside.

2 Heat wok on high heat for 1 minute. Swirl in oil. Add bok choy and stir-fry for about 1 minute, until softened. Add garlic mixture and stir-fry for about 1 minute, until tender-crisp. Remove from heat and stir in onions. Serve immediately.

NUTRIENTS	CALORIES	FAT	CARBOHYDRATE	PROTEIN	FIBER
per serving	86	7.3 g	4.8 g	1.9 g	1.4 g

Sheet Pan Broccoli and Cauliflower

MAKES 6 SERVINGS

SERVING SIZE: ABOUT 1 CUP (250 ML)

Sheet-pan recipes are made for weeknights. There is minimal mess, and once you get the sheet pan in the oven there is not much else to do— except wait for your delicious food to be cooked to perfection.

Preheat oven to 400°F (200°C)

TIP
Get creative with your sheet pan vegetables. Add a sprinkle of freshly grated Parmesan cheese, a squeeze of lemon juice or a handful of toasted pine nuts to your vegetables after they come out of the oven.

3 tbsp	olive oil	45 mL
4	cloves garlic, thinly sliced	4
½ tsp	salt	2 mL
¼ tsp	freshly ground black pepper	1 mL
⅛ tsp	hot pepper flakes	0.5 mL
1	head broccoli, cut into florets	1
1	head cauliflower, cut into florets	1

1. In a large bowl, whisk together the oil, garlic, salt, black pepper and pepper flakes. Add the broccoli and cauliflower florets and toss to evenly coat.

2. Place the broccoli and cauliflower in a single layer on a sheet pan. Roast in the preheated oven until browned on the edges, 20 to 25 minutes.

NUTRIENTS per serving	CALORIES	FAT	CARBOHYDRATE	PROTEIN	FIBER
	132	7.5 g	14.4 g	5.7 g	5.5 g

Brussels Sprouts with Almond Thyme Butter

Almond thyme butter transforms simple steamed Brussels sprouts from ordinary to extraordinary. Use the luscious leftover butter to add excitement to other steamed vegetables.

Food processor

TIPS

To prepare Brussels sprouts for this recipe: Trim and cut a shallow X in the base of each sprout. Reserve any leaves that fall off in a separate pile.

To toast almonds, cook them in a dry skillet over medium heat, stirring often, for about 3 minutes or until golden and aromatic.

1 lb	Brussels sprouts, trimmed (see Tips)	500 g
⅓ cup	slivered almonds, toasted, divided (see Tips)	75 mL
¼ cup	unsalted butter or non-dairy alternative, softened	60 mL
2 tsp	finely grated lemon zest	10 mL
½ tsp	fresh thyme leaves	2 mL
1 tsp	liquid honey or vegan alternative	5 mL
½ tsp	kosher or coarse sea salt	2 mL

1 In a covered steamer basket over boiling water 1 inch (2.5 cm) deep, cook Brussels sprouts for 10 to 12 minutes, until tender but firm, adding loose leaves midway through the cooking time.

2 Meanwhile, in bowl of food processor fitted with the metal blade, process all but 1 tbsp (15 mL) almonds until finely ground but not pasty. Add butter, lemon zest, thyme, honey and salt. Pulse a few times, just until combined; you should end up with ½ cup (125 mL).

3 Remove steamer basket from heat and set aside for 1 minute to allow Brussels sprouts to drain and release steam. Transfer sprouts to a serving dish and add almond butter to taste (you will have some left over); toss to coat evenly. Scatter reserved almonds overtop. Serve immediately.

Variation

Pecan Thyme Butter: Substitute an equal amount of coarsely chopped toasted pecans for the almonds.

Brussels Sprouts

Brussels sprouts are high in vitamin C. Cooking can often lower a vegetable's vitamin C content. To maintain as much vitamin C as possible, eating these veggies raw or lightly steamed is often best.

NUTRIENTS per serving	CALORIES	FAT	CARBOHYDRATE	PROTEIN	FIBER
	294	23.8 g	16.9 g	9 g	7.4 g

Stir-Fried Brussels Sprouts

MAKES 4 TO 6 SERVINGS

¼ cup	chicken broth	50 mL
1 tbsp	soy sauce	15 mL
2 tsp	hoisin sauce	10 mL
1 tsp	cornstarch	5 mL
2 tbsp	vegetable oil	30 mL
2 cups	Brussels sprouts, trimmed and halved	500 mL
½ cup	chopped onion	125 mL
2	cloves garlic, minced	2
2 tsp	minced gingerroot	10 mL
	Salt and freshly ground black pepper to taste	

Combine broth, soy sauce, hoisin sauce and cornstarch; set aside.

In a wok or large skillet, heat oil over medium-high heat.

Stir-fry Brussels sprouts and onion, covering pan between stirrings, for about 8 minutes, or until vegetables are browned and sprouts are almost tender.

Add garlic, ginger, salt and pepper; stir-fry for 1 minute.

Stir broth mixture, add to pan and stir-fry until vegetables are coated and sauce is slightly thickened, about oil and almonds.

NUTRIENTS	CALORIES	FAT	CARBOHYDRATE	PROTEIN	FIBER
per serving	82	5.7 g	6.9 g	2 g	1.7 g

Sautéed Red Chard with Lemon and Pine Nuts

MAKES 2 SERVINGS

This colorful and easy addition to the dinner table makes eating your greens a pleasure, not a chore. Serve it over brown rice or whole grains.

TIP

To prepare the chard for this recipe: Trim, separating stems and thick center ribs from the leaves. Using a sharp knife, cut stems and ribs into ½-inch (1 cm) pieces. Chop the leaves coarsely. Set aside in separate piles.

2 tbsp	extra-virgin olive oil	30 mL
2 tbsp	pine nuts	30 mL
1	small bunch red chard (12 oz/375 g), trimmed, leaves chopped and stems cut into ½-inch (1 cm) pieces (see Tip)	1
2	large cloves garlic, chopped	2
½ tsp	kosher or coarse sea salt	2 mL
⅛ tsp	freshly ground black pepper	0.5 mL
2 tsp	freshly squeezed lemon juice (see Tips)	10 mL
½ cup	shredded smoked Gouda (2 oz/60 g), optional	125 mL

1. In a large skillet over medium heat, heat oil until shimmery. Fry pine nuts, stirring often, for about 2 minutes, until golden. Using a slotted spoon, transfer nuts to a small bowl.

2. Add chard stems to same skillet and cook over medium heat, stirring often, for about 5 minutes, until softened. Stir in garlic for 20 seconds. Add chard leaves, salt and pepper and cook, stirring often, for about 5 minutes, until leaves are wilted and tender and stems are tender-crisp. Stir in lemon juice and remove from heat. Stir in pine nuts.

3. Transfer to a microwave-safe serving bowl or individual plates. Sprinkle with cheese (if using). Heat in microwave on High for 1 minute or until cheese is molten.

NUTRIENTS	CALORIES	FAT	CARBOHYDRATE	PROTEIN	FIBER
per serving	214	19.7 g	8.9 g	4.4 g	3.1 g

Eggplant with Tomatoes and Cumin

MAKES 6 SERVINGS

SERVING SIZE: ⅔ CUP (150 ML)

This dish is perfect for meal prepping and reheating, especially with the tomato-based sauce.

TIP

When choosing eggplants, pick them up. They should feel heavy in your hand. The skin should be smooth and shiny, and when you press your fingers, it should feel slightly firm. Choose small- to medium-size eggplant, as the larger sizes tend to be bitter.

2 tbsp	olive oil	30 mL
2	cloves garlic, minced	2
1	eggplant, diced into 2-inch (5 cm) cubes	1
1¾ cups	no-salt-added canned diced tomatoes, with juice	425 mL
1 tsp	ground cumin	5 mL
1 tsp	smoked paprika	5 mL
¼ tsp	salt	1 mL
⅛ tsp	ground black pepper	0.5 mL

1. In a large sauté pan, heat the olive oil over medium heat. When the oil is shimmering, add the garlic and cook until fragrant, 30 seconds. Add the eggplant and cook until softened, 10 minutes, turning occasionally.

2. Add the diced tomatoes with juice, cumin, smoked paprika, salt and pepper and toss to combine. Raise the heat to high and bring the mixture to a boil. Reduce the heat to medium-low and simmer, covered, until the flavors combine, 10 minutes.

3. **TO STORE:** In each of six containers, add ⅔ cup (150 mL) of the eggplant mixture. Cover and refrigerate for up to 4 days or freeze for up to 2 months.

4. **TO SERVE:** If frozen, thaw in the refrigerator overnight. To reheat, microwave uncovered on High for 1 minute. Allow 2 minutes for the heat to distribute before removing the container from the microwave. Serve warm.

NUTRIENTS per serving	CALORIES 87.99	FAT 4.79 g	CARBOHYDRATE 8.84 g	PROTEIN 2.21 g	FIBER 4.22 g

Garlicky Okra

MAKES 6 TO 8 SERVINGS

The trick to removing the sliminess of okra is simply to sauté them, stirring gently. This simple recipe is both tasty and healthy. Always look for young tender okra, as the bigger pods are tough.

TIP

Kokum is the thick black skin of a sour tropical plum-like fruit, used to add an element of tartness. If not using kokum, add additional 1 tsp (5 mL) mango powder.

2 lbs	okra	1 kg
3 tbsp	oil	45 mL
16	cloves garlic, sliced and crushed	16
¼ tsp	asafetida (hing)	1 mL
2 cups	chopped onions	500 mL
4	2-inch (5 cm) long green chiles, preferably serranos, halved lengthwise	4
18	kokum, optional (see Tip)	18
1 tsp	salt or to taste	5 mL
1 tsp	mango powder (amchur)	5 mL

1. Rinse okra and pat dry. Cut into ½-inch (1 cm) pieces. Set aside.

2. In a skillet, heat oil over medium heat. Add garlic and asafetida and sauté until garlic is golden, about 2 minutes.

3. Add onions and sauté until golden, 7 to 8 minutes.

4. Add chiles and sauté for 2 minutes. Add kokum, if using, and sauté for 1 minute.

5. Add okra and mix well. Sauté, stirring frequently, until there is no more sliminess, 10 to 15 minutes. Adjust heat to prevent burning but maintain a gentle sizzle at all times. If okra is not completely cooked, add 1 tbsp (15 mL) water. Reduce heat to low. Cover and cook until tender. Shake pan periodically to prevent burning.

6. Remove from heat, sprinkle with salt and mix. Sprinkle mango powder over top. Serve as a side dish.

What Is Asafetida?

Asafetida (or asafoetida), often known as hing, comes from the roots of ferula plants. The dried powder is commonly used as a seasoning in Indian cooking and is known for its anti-inflammatory and antioxidant properties.

NUTRIENTS	CALORIES	FAT	CARBOHYDRATE	PROTEIN	FIBER
per serving	131	6.4 g	17.9 g	3.5 g	5.3 g

Garlic Sautéed Spinach

MAKES 4 SERVINGS

SERVING SIZE: ABOUT ½ CUP (125 ML)

Garlic not only adds an aromatic flavor to dishes, but it also comes with an array of good-for-you nutrients. One clove of garlic contains calcium and several B vitamins. Garlic also has the plant chemical allicin, shown to have antibacterial properties.

TIP
Remember to drain your thawed spinach before cooking. This will prevent the spinach from becoming wet and soggy.

2 tbsp	olive oil or canola oil	30 mL
3	cloves garlic, minced	3
10-oz	package frozen chopped spinach, thawed and well drained	300 g
¼ tsp	salt	1 mL
⅛ tsp	freshly ground black pepper	0.5 mL

1 Heat the oil in a large skillet over medium heat. When the oil is shimmering, add the garlic and cook until fragrant, 30 seconds. Add the spinach and cook until warmed through, 5 minutes. Sprinkle with the salt and pepper and toss to combine.

NUTRIENTS per serving	CALORIES 84	FAT 7.2 g	CARBOHYDRATE 3.8 g	PROTEIN 2.7 g	FIBER 2.1 g

Winter Greens with Split Yellow Peas / Saag aur Channa Dal

MAKES 8 SERVINGS

Rich in nutrients and equally tasty, this unusual combination is a favorite winter dishes when turnip and mustard greens are at their freshest.

TIP

Greens, when cooked, reduce drastically in volume, so a little bit more or a little bit less will not change the dish.

1 cup	split yellow peas (channa dal)	250 mL
½ tsp	turmeric	2 mL
2½ tsp	salt or to taste, divided	12 mL
6 to 7 cups	spinach, rinsed and chopped (see Tip)	1.5 to 1.75 L
6 to 7 cups	turnip greens, rinsed and chopped	1.5 to 1.75 L
6 to 7 cups	mustard or collard greens, rinsed and chopped	1.5 to 1.75 L
2 tbsp	oil	30 mL
2 tbsp	slivered peeled gingerroot	30 mL
1 tbsp	minced green chiles, preferably serranos	15 mL
2 tbsp	dark mustard seeds, coarsely pounded	30 mL
1 tbsp	cumin seeds	15 mL
1½ tsp	salt or to taste	7 mL
2 tbsp	freshly squeezed lime or lemon juice or to taste	30 mL

1. Clean and pick through dal for any small stones and grit. Rinse several times in cold water until water is fairly clear. Soak in 2½ cups (625 mL) water in a saucepan for 15 minutes.

2. Bring dal to a boil over medium heat. Reduce heat to low. Stir in turmeric and boil gently, partially covered, until dal is soft but not mushy and water is absorbed, 20 to 25 minutes. Add 1 tsp (5 mL) of the salt in the last 5 minutes of cooking. Set aside.

3. In a large pot, combine spinach, turnip and mustard greens and 2 tbsp (30 mL) water. Cover and cook over low heat, until water is absorbed, about 5 minutes.

4. Meanwhile, in a large skillet, heat oil over medium heat. Add ginger and chiles and sauté for 1 minute. Add mustard and cumin and sauté, stirring continuously, for 2 minutes.

5. Add spinach mixture, dal and remaining salt. Mix well and heat through. Add lime juice to taste. Serve with Indian bread.

NUTRIENTS	CALORIES	FAT	CARBOHYDRATE	PROTEIN	FIBER
per serving	165	5.7 g	22.7 g	8.7 g	9.2 g

Sautéed Zucchini with Lemon and Pine Nuts

MAKES 4 SERVINGS

SERVING SIZE: ¾ CUP (175 ML)

This will make a wonderful addition to your side dish repertoire.

TIP
Swap the zucchini for yellow squash or use a combination of both to add color.

3 tbsp	pine nuts	45 mL
2 tbsp	olive oil or canola oil	30 mL
1	clove garlic, minced	1
3	medium zucchini, sliced into 1-inch (2.5 cm) rounds	3
½ tsp	salt	2 mL
¼ tsp	freshly ground black pepper	1 mL
	Juice of 1 lemon	

1 Place the pine nuts in a medium skillet over medium-low heat. Toast the pine nuts, stirring regularly, until slightly browned, 3 minutes. Spoon the pine nuts into a small bowl; set aside to slightly cool.

2 Heat the oil in the same skillet over medium heat. When the oil is shimmering, add the garlic and cook until fragrant, 30 seconds. Add the zucchini and cook until slightly softened, 10 minutes. Add the salt, pepper and lemon juice and toss to combine.

3 Place the zucchini in a serving dish and sprinkle with the toasted pine nuts. Serve warm.

Make Ahead
Toast the pine nuts up to 1 week in advance and store in a sealed container in a cool, dry place until ready to use.

NUTRIENTS	CALORIES	FAT	CARBOHYDRATE	PROTEIN	FIBER
per serving	133	11.6 g	7.1 g	2.9 g	2.2 g

Ginger and Orange Braised Carrots

MAKES 6 SERVINGS

Here, carrots are briefly pressure cooked, then simmered down in orange juice and butter for a sweet and tender braised finish with bright citrus notes.

Instant Pot

TIPS

A 1-inch (2.5 cm) square piece of ginger will yield about 4 tsp (20 mL) grated.

For a slightly spicier, herbal tone, substitute ½ tsp (2 mL) ground cardamom for the ginger. Omit the lemon juice.

This recipe can easily be doubled for a large gathering.

1½ lbs	carrots, cut diagonally into ½-inch (1 cm) thick slices	750 g
4 tsp	grated gingerroot	20 mL
¾ cup	water	175 mL
½ cup	orange juice, divided	125 mL
3 tbsp	butter, softened, divided	45 mL
	Salt and freshly ground black pepper	
1½ tsp	freshly squeezed lemon juice (optional)	7 mL
	Chopped fresh parsley (optional)	

1 In the inner pot of the Instant Pot, combine carrots, ginger, water, ¼ cup (60 mL) orange juice and 1 tbsp (15 mL) butter.

2 Close and lock the lid and turn the steam release handle to Sealing. Set your Instant Pot to pressure cook on High for 2 minutes.

3 When the cooking time is done, press Cancel and turn the steam release handle to Venting. When the float valve drops down, remove the lid. Drain carrots.

4 Set your Instant Pot to sauté on More. When the display says Hot, add the remaining butter and heat until melted. Stir in carrots and the remaining orange juice; cook, stirring gently occasionally, for 3 minutes or until liquid has evaporated and carrots are fork-tender.

5 Transfer carrots to a serving bowl and season to taste with salt and pepper. If desired, drizzle with lemon juice and sprinkle with parsley.

NUTRIENTS	CALORIES	FAT	CARBOHYDRATE	PROTEIN	FIBER
per serving	108	6.1 g	13.3 g	1.3 g	3.2 g

Honey Roasted Carrots

MAKES 6 SERVINGS

SERVING SIZE: ¾ CUP (175 ML)

Vegetable side dishes don't have to be complicated or have a long list of ingredients. The baby carrots needed for this recipe require no prep. Just toss them with honey, parsley and olive oil, and they're ready for the oven. It really doesn't get easier than that!

Preheat oven to 400°F (200°C)

Nonstick cooking spray		
2 tbsp	olive oil or canola oil	30 mL
2 tbsp	honey	30 mL
1 tsp	dried parsley	5 mL
1 lb	baby carrots	500 g

1 Coat a baking sheet with nonstick cooking spray.

2 In a large bowl, whisk together the oil, honey and parsley. Add the carrots and toss to coat.

3 Place the carrots in a single layer on the prepared sheet pan. Roast in the preheated oven until softened and slightly browned, 25 to 30 minutes.

NUTRIENTS per serving	CALORIES	FAT	CARBOHYDRATE	PROTEIN	FIBER
	92	4.7 g	13.1 g	0.7 g	2.1 g

Oven-Roasted Mixed Veggies

MAKES 2 TO 3 SERVINGS

This colorful vegetable combination is a snap to prepare. If I have any leftovers, I include them in a salad for lunch. Baby potatoes can be replaced with sweet potatoes, cut in ½-inch (1 cm) pieces. Serve with cold roast chicken, cold ham or deli meats.

8 oz	baby potatoes, halved (quartered if largish)	250 g
1 tbsp	olive oil	15 mL
½ tsp	salt	2 mL
¼ tsp	black pepper	1 mL
1	small zucchini, halved lengthwise and cut in ½-inch (1 cm) pieces	1
½	red bell pepper, seeded and cut in ½-inch (1 cm) pieces	½
8 oz	thin asparagus, tough ends removed, cut in 2-inch (5 cm) lengths	250 g
4 oz	green beans, trimmed and halved crosswise	125 g

1 Arrange potatoes on parchment- or foil-lined oven pan. Add oil, salt and pepper, toss and turn potatoes to coat with oil, then arrange in a single layer. Roast in preheated 425°F (220°C) toaster oven for 12 minutes.

2 Add zucchini, red pepper, asparagus and green beans to oven pan. Toss to coat all vegetables with oil. Roast for 15 to 18 minutes, or until all vegetables are tender.

NUTRIENTS	CALORIES	FAT	CARBOHYDRATE	PROTEIN	FIBER
per serving	172	6 g	27.1 g	6 g	6.6 g

Oven-Baked Sweet Potato Fries with Curry Mayo

MAKES 8 SERVINGS

Oven-baking sweet potato fries lowers the fat and calories while maintaining all the flavor. The curry mayo was a real hit with our taste testers.

Preheat oven to 425°F (220°C)

Baking sheet, lined with foil

TIPS

Cut the potatoes to a uniform size and shape to facilitate even cooking.

Kids can get involved by making the curry mayo.

If you serve these fries without the curry mayo, you'll reduce the fat content per serving by a third.

Jessica Kelly, Dietitian, Ontario

SWEET POTATO FRIES

1½ lbs	sweet potatoes, peeled and cut into ½-inch (1 cm) thick spears	750 g
¼ cup	canola or olive oil	60 mL
1 tsp	ground cumin	5 mL
½ tsp	sea salt (optional)	2 mL

CURRY MAYO

¼ cup	light mayonnaise	60 mL
1 tsp	curry powder	5 mL
1 tsp	liquid honey	5 mL

1 **FRIES:** In a large bowl, combine sweet potatoes, oil and cumin, tossing until fries are well coated. Spread in a single layer on prepared baking sheet. Bake in preheated oven for 15 minutes. Flip potatoes over and bake for 15 minutes or until browned and tender. Transfer potatoes to a plate lined with paper towels and sprinkle with sea salt (if using).

2 **MAYO:** Meanwhile, in a small bowl, combine mayonnaise, curry powder and honey. Cover and refrigerate until ready to use.

3 Serve fries with curry mayo for dipping.

Variation

Use 1 tsp (5 mL) paprika and 1 tsp (5 mL) chili powder in place of cumin. Or use 1 tsp (5 mL) ground cinnamon and 2 tbsp (30 mL) chopped fresh rosemary.

NUTRIENTS	CALORIES	FAT	CARBOHYDRATE	PROTEIN	FIBER
per serving	146	9.5 g	15 g	1 g	2 g

Roasted Sweet Potatoes

MAKES 8 SERVINGS

SERVING SIZE ½ CUP (125 ML)

These lightly seasoned oven-roasted sweet potatoes are so scrumptious that you'll forget they are heart healthy. This side dish is sure to become part of your regular meal prepping repertoire.

Preheat oven to 400°F (200°C)

Rimmed baking sheet lined with parchment paper

TIP

If you prefer, swap the sweet potatoes for russet potatoes.

2 tbsp	olive oil	30 mL
1 tsp	ground cumin	5 mL
½ tsp	chili powder	2 mL
¼ tsp	salt	1 mL
3	sweet potatoes (2 lbs/1 kg), peeled and cut into 1-inch (2.5 cm) dice	3

1. In a large bowl, whisk together the oil, cumin, chili powder and salt. Add the potatoes and toss to evenly coat.

2. Place the sweet potatoes in a single layer on the prepared baking sheet. Roast, tossing halfway through, until the potatoes are fork-tender, 20 to 25 minutes.

3. **TO STORE:** In each of eight containers, add ½ cup (125 mL) of the sweet potatoes. Cover and refrigerate for up to 4 days or freeze for up to 2 months.

4. **TO SERVE:** If frozen, thaw in the refrigerator overnight. To reheat, microwave uncovered on High for 60 to 90 seconds. Allow 2 minutes for the heat to distribute before removing the container from the microwave. Serve warm.

NUTRIENTS	CALORIES	FAT	CARBOHYDRATE	PROTEIN	FIBER
per serving	106.05	2.64 g	19.39 g	1.55 g	2.97 g

Buttery Garlic Mashed Potatoes

MAKES 4 SERVINGS

Instant Pot

Steamer basket

TIPS

You can substitute small yellow-fleshed potatoes, as long as they weigh about 1½ lbs (750 g) total. Reduce the pressure cooking time to 5 minutes. You don't need to peel the potatoes before mashing them.

If your steamer basket doesn't have legs, place a steam rack in the pot first and place the steamer basket on the rack.

Mash potatoes just until they are your desired consistency and everything is combined. Do not overmash.

4	russet potatoes (about 1½ lbs/750 g total), peeled and cut into 1½-inch (4 cm) pieces	4
5 tbsp	butter, softened, divided	75 mL
3	cloves garlic, minced	3
¼ cup	ready-to-use reduced-sodium chicken broth or low-sodium chicken stock	60 mL
¼ cup	heavy or whipping (35%) cream (approx.)	60 mL
	Salt and freshly ground black pepper	

1 Add 1 cup (250 mL) hot water to the inner pot of the Instant Pot and place the steamer basket in the pot (see Tip). Place potatoes in the basket.

2 Close and lock the lid and turn the steam release handle to Sealing. Set your Instant Pot to pressure cook on High for 8 minutes.

3 When the cooking time is done, press Cancel and turn the steam release handle to Venting. When the float valve drops down, remove the lid. The potatoes should be fork-tender. (If more cooking time is needed, continue pressure cooking on High for 1 minute.) Remove steamer basket and set aside. Discard water.

4 Set your Instant Pot to sauté on Normal. When the display says Hot, add 2 tbsp (30 mL) butter and heat until melted. Add garlic and cook, stirring, for 1 minute or until fragrant. Add potatoes and the remaining butter; start mashing potatoes. When butter is absorbed, add broth, mashing until combined. Press Cancel.

5 Gradually add cream, mashing, until potatoes are your desired consistency. (Use only as much cream as is needed to reach that consistency.) Season to taste with salt and pepper. Transfer to a serving bowl. Serve immediately.

NUTRIENTS	CALORIES	FAT	CARBOHYDRATE	PROTEIN	FIBER
per serving	313	20 g	31 g	4.3 g	3.6 g

Crushed Potatoes with Black Sesame Seeds / Kalay Tilwalle Aloo

MAKES 6 TO 8 SERVINGS

These potatoes can be served hot or at room temperature. Take them on a picnic to replace potato salad and you'll win kudos.

2½ lbs	small red or white new potatoes	1.25 kg
3 tbsp	mustard oil	45 mL
2½ tsp	black sesame seeds	12 mL
2 tsp	hot pepper flakes	10 mL
¾ tsp	turmeric	4 mL
2 tsp	salt or to taste	10 mL
¼ cup	freshly squeezed lime or lemon juice	60 mL
2 tbsp	cilantro, chopped	30 mL

1 Place potatoes in a large saucepan filled three-quarters full of water. Bring to a boil over high heat. Reduce heat to medium and cook just until tender, 12 to 14 minutes.

2 Drain and let cool slightly. Press each potato between palms to "crush," by applying gentle pressure, keeping potato intact. This exposes parts of the inside of the potato to the spices and creates a crusty potato.

3 In a large skillet, heat oil over high heat until almost smoking. Remove from heat and let cool for 1 minute. Return skillet to medium heat. Add sesame seeds, hot pepper flakes and turmeric and sauté for 1 minute.

4 Add potatoes and salt and mix well. Drizzle 1 tbsp (15 mL) water around edges of pan. Cover, reduce heat to low and cook for about 10 minutes, stirring every 3 to 4 minutes. Shake pan periodically. Potatoes should be slightly crusty and coated in masala.

5 Remove from heat and pour lime juice over top. Stir to mix. Garnish with cilantro. Serve with an Indian bread.

NUTRIENTS	CALORIES	FAT	CARBOHYDRATE	PROTEIN	FIBER
per serving	188	6.7 g	29.6 g	3.6 g	3.7 g

Red Potatoes with Chives

Red potatoes are small to medium in size and have thin red skin and white flesh. The texture of these spuds is creamy and smooth with a subtly sweet flavor. These potatoes work well roasted (like in this recipe) or mashed, or try them in soups, stews and salads.

Preheat oven to 425°F (220°C)

Rimmed baking sheet lined with parchment paper

2 tbsp	olive oil	30 mL
2	cloves garlic, minced	2
1 tsp	dried chives	5 mL
¼ tsp	salt	1 mL
¼ tsp	ground black pepper	1 mL
2 lbs	small red potatoes, thoroughly cleaned and dried	1 kg

1 In a large bowl, whisk together the oil, garlic, chives, salt and pepper. Add the potatoes and toss to combine.

2 Place the potatoes in a single layer on the prepared baking sheet and bake, tossing halfway through, until tender, 30 minutes. Remove from the oven and let cool for 10 minutes.

3 **TO STORE:** In each of 10 containers, add ½ cup (125 mL) of the potatoes. Cover and refrigerate for up to 4 days or freeze for up to 2 months.

4 **TO SERVE:** If frozen, thaw in the refrigerator overnight. To reheat, microwave uncovered on High for 90 seconds. Allow 2 minutes for the heat to distribute before removing the container from the microwave. Serve warm.

NUTRIENTS	CALORIES	FAT	CARBOHYDRATE	PROTEIN	FIBER
per serving	82.20	2.15 g	14.58 g	1.75 g	1.56 g

Israeli Couscous and Mushrooms

SERVING SIZE: ¾ CUP (175 ML)

Couscous isn't a grain but rather a combination of semolina wheat and water, which makes it more like pasta. There are several types of couscous, including small Moroccan couscous (about three times the size of cornmeal) and the large Israeli couscous (also called pearled couscous). This recipe uses the Israeli type, which takes less than 10 minutes to cook.

TIP

For a nutrient boost, use whole wheat Israeli couscous.

1 tbsp	olive oil or canola oil	15 mL
1	onion, chopped	1
1	clove garlic, minced	1
8 oz	cremini mushrooms, thinly sliced	250 g
1 cup	Israeli couscous	250 mL
1¼ cups	reduced-sodium ready-to-use vegetable broth	310 mL
¼ tsp	dried dillweed	1 mL
¼ tsp	salt	1 mL
⅛ tsp	freshly ground black pepper	0.5 mL

1 Heat the oil in a medium skillet over medium heat. When the oil is shimmering, add the onion and garlic and cook, stirring occasionally, until the onion is translucent and the garlic is fragrant, 3 minutes. Add the mushrooms and cook, stirring occasionally, until softened, 5 minutes.

2 Add the couscous, broth, dillweed, salt and pepper and bring the mixture to a boil. Reduce the heat to medium-low, cover and simmer until the couscous is cooked al dente, 8 minutes. Fluff with a fork before serving.

NUTRIENTS	CALORIES	FAT	CARBOHYDRATE	PROTEIN	FIBER
per serving	225	3.9 g	39.8 g	7.9 g	3.4 g

Brown Rice with Peas and Carrots

MAKES 4 SERVINGS

SERVING SIZE: 1 CUP (250 ML)

Brown rice is considered a whole grain because the bran and germ, which are removed in white rice, are left intact. This means that you get more nutrients like filling fiber, hunger-fighting protein and energy-boosting B vitamins. Brown rice does take longer to cook than some other grains, but it is simple to prepare.

TIP

Bay leaves impart a delicious flavor to dishes but should be added toward the beginning of a recipe so the flavor has time to seep into your dish. Don't forget to discard the leaf before eating.

1 tbsp	olive oil	15 mL
1	onion, chopped	1
2	cloves garlic, minced	2
2	carrots, shredded	2
1 cup	frozen peas, thawed	250 mL
1 cup	long-grain brown rice	250 mL
2 cups	reduced-sodium ready-to-use vegetable or chicken broth	500 mL
2	bay leaves	2
½ tsp	salt	2 mL
¼ tsp	freshly ground black pepper	1 mL

1 Heat the oil in a medium saucepan over medium heat. When the oil is shimmering, add the onion and garlic and cook, stirring occasionally, until the onion is translucent and the garlic is fragrant, 3 minutes. Add the carrots and peas and cook, stirring occasionally, until softened, 5 minutes. Add the rice and cook, stirring occasionally, for 2 to 3 minutes.

2 Add the broth and bay leaves to the saucepan, raise the heat to high and bring to a boil. Lower the heat to medium-low and simmer, covered, stirring occasionally, until the rice is tender, about 40 minutes. Drain any excess water. Transfer the rice to a large bowl, fluff with a fork and stir in the salt and pepper. Remove the bay leaves and discard.

NUTRIENTS per serving	CALORIES 268	FAT 4.2 g	CARBOHYDRATE 50.7 g	PROTEIN 6.6 g	FIBER 4.6 g

Cayenne-Spiked Apricot and Nuts Pulao

The spicy, sweet taste of this rich dish, combined with the texture of nuts and dried fruit, makes it a fabulous party dish. It is good with meat or chicken curry but equally wonderful with roast chicken or turkey.

TIP

True basmati rice comes from the foothills of the Himalayas. There is rice available in the bulk bins of some supermarkets that is marked basmati but it is usually from California and does not work in these recipes. Be sure to use only Indian or Pakistani basmati rice.

1½ cups	Indian basmati rice (see Tip)	375 mL
½ tsp	saffron threads	2 mL
½ cup	granulated sugar	125 mL
1	stick cinnamon, about 3 inches (7.5 cm) long	1
4	whole cloves	4
2 tbsp	cayenne pepper or to taste	30 mL
¼ cup	freshly squeezed lime or lemon juice	60 mL
½ cup	dried apricots	125 mL
½ cup	whole blanched almonds	125 mL
½ cup	walnut or pecan halves	125 mL
2 tbsp	oil	30 mL
1½ cups	thinly sliced onions (lengthwise slices)	375 mL
1½ tsp	salt	7 mL

1. Place rice in a bowl with plenty of cold water and swish vigorously with fingers. Drain. Repeat process 4 or 5 times until water is fairly clear. Cover with 3 to 4 inches (7.5 to 10 cm) cold water and soak for 15 minutes or for up to 2 hours.

2. In a bowl, soak saffron in ¼ cup (50 mL) very hot water for 15 minutes.

3. In a saucepan, cook sugar, ½ cup (125 mL) water, cinnamon, cloves and cayenne over medium heat until mixture is bubbly and syrupy, 5 to 7 minutes. Stir in lime juice. Mix in apricots, almonds and walnuts or pecans. Set aside.

4. In a large saucepan, heat oil over medium-high heat. Add onions and sauté until golden, 6 to 8 minutes.

5. Drain rice and stir into onions. Sauté for 2 minutes. Stir in nut mixture and saffron with liquid. Add 1¾ cups (425 mL) cold water and salt. Cover and bring to a boil. Reduce heat to as low as possible and cook, without peeking, for 25 minutes. Remove from heat and set lid slightly ajar to allow steam to escape. Let rest for 5 minutes for rice to firm up. Fluff gently with fork. Gently spoon onto a platter to serve.

NUTRIENTS per serving	CALORIES 349	FAT 13.2 g	CARBOHYDRATE 54.5 g	PROTEIN 6.2 g	FIBER 4.9 g

Simple Rice Pilaf

1 tbsp	butter	15 mL
¼ cup	finely chopped onion	50 mL
1 cup	long-grain white rice	250 mL
2 cups	chicken broth	500 mL
	Salt and freshly ground	
	Black pepper to taste	

In a saucepan, melt butter over medium heat.

Sauté onion until tender.

Add rice, stirring to coat with butter.

Add broth, salt and pepper, stirring briefly to moisten rice.

Bring to a boil, reduce heat, cover and simmer for 15 to 20 minutes, or until liquid is absorbed and rice is tender. (Do not stir rice when checking for doneness.)

Remove from heat and let stand, covered, for 5 minutes. Fluff with a fork.

Variation

Rice Pilaf with Walnuts: Follow recipe for Simple Rice Pilaf, but while rice is cooking, toast ⅓ cup (75 mL) chopped walnuts in 1 tbsp (15 mL) walnut oil. Toss with the rice while fluffing.

NUTRIENTS	CALORIES	FAT	CARBOHYDRATE	PROTEIN	FIBER
per serving	166	2.7 g	31.4 g	3.3 g	1.2 g

Quinoa Pilaf

NUTRITION TIP
The recommended daily fiber intake varies depending on age and sex. Adult women should target 25 grams of fiber per day. Adult men should target 38 grams of fiber per day.

1½ tbsp	canola oil	22 mL
2 tbsp	minced onion	30 mL
2 tbsp	diced celery	30 mL
2 tbsp	diced carrot	30 mL
1 cup	quinoa, rinsed in several changes of water	250 mL
2 cups	hot vegetable or chicken broth	500 mL
	Salt and freshly ground black pepper to taste	

In a heavy saucepan, heat oil over medium heat.

Sauté onion, celery and carrot until tender.

Add quinoa and cook, stirring, until grains separate.

Add broth, salt and pepper; bring to a simmer.

Reduce heat, cover and simmer for about 20 minutes, or until liquid is absorbed and quinoa is tender. Fluff with a fork.

Quinoa
Quinoa offers 5 grams of fiber per cooked 1-cup serving.

NUTRIENTS per serving	CALORIES	FAT	CARBOHYDRATE	PROTEIN	FIBER
	171	6.5 g	23 g	5.5 g	2.6 g

Tabbouleh with Lentils

1 cup	dried brown lentils	250 mL
5 cups	water, divided	1.25 mL
¾ cup	medium-grain bulgur, rinsed thoroughly	175 mL
½ tsp	salt	2 mL
Pinch	ground allspice	Pinch
3	green onions, finely chopped	3
2	cloves garlic, minced	2
1	cucumber, peeled, seeded and diced	1
1 cup	diced seeded tomato	250 mL
¼ cup	chopped fresh mint	60 mL
¼ cup	chopped fresh Italian (flat-leaf) parsley	60 mL
¼ cup	freshly squeezed lemon juice	60 mL
¼ cup	olive oil	60 mL
	Lettuce leaves	
	Lemon wedges	

Boil lentils in 4 cups (1 L) of the water for 40 minutes; drain.

Combine bulgur and lentils in a large bowl.

Bring the remaining water, salt and allspice to a boil; add to bulgur mixture and let stand until water is absorbed.

Toss with green onions, garlic, cucumber, tomato, mint, parsley, lemon juice and olive oil.

Serve on lettuce leaves, garnished with lemon wedges.

NUTRIENTS	CALORIES	FAT	CARBOHYDRATE	PROTEIN	FIBER
per serving	328	11.7 g	46.2 g	13.2 g	8 g

Library and Archives Canada Cataloguing in Publication
Title: The complete gout management & nutrition guide : empowering strategies for
better health / Diana Girnita, MD, PhD, FACR with Doug Cook, RD, MHSc.
Other titles: Gout management & nutrition guide
Names: Girnita, Diana, author. | Cook, Doug, 1964- author.
Description: Includes index.
Identifiers: Canadiana 20240346653 | ISBN 9780778807230 (softcover)
Subjects: LCSH: Gout. | LCSH: Gout—Diet therapy. | LCSH: Gout—Treatment.
Classification: LCC RC629 .G57 2024 | DDC 616.7/220654—dc23

■ *Dietitians of Canada Cook! 275 Recipes Celebrate Food from Field to Table,* by Mary Sue Waisman
Great Grains, Fruit and Nut Granola with Honey and Almond Butter
Cornmeal Crêpes with Avocado Filling
Brined and Tender Lemon Roast Chicken
Pasta with Chicken and Vegetable Sauce
Legume and Veggie Burgers
Roasted Lemon Asparagus
Oven-Baked Sweet Potato Fries with Curry Mayo
Citrus Fennel Slaw

■ *150 Best Toaster Oven Recipes,* by Linda Stephen
Spanish Potato Frittata
Mushroom Bread Cups
Chicken Turnovers
Date Orange Muffins
Oven-Roasted Mixed Veggies

■ *175 Best Instant Pot Recipes: For Your Programmable Electric Pressure Cooker,* by Marilyn Haugen
Apple Yogurt Chia Power Breakfast
Maple Cinnamon Breakfast Quinoa
Forbidden Black Rice with Coconut
Ginger Pumpkin Soup
Chicken and Wild Rice Soup

All published by Robert Rose

■ *5-Ingredient Instant Pot Cookbook: 150 Easy, Quick and Delicious Meals,* by Marilyn Haugen
Peanut Butter and Banana Oatmeal
Ginger and Orange Braised Carrots
Buttery Garlic Mashed Potatoes

■ *The Wok and Skillet Cookbook: 300 Recipes for Stir-Frys and Noodles,* by Nancie McDermott
Tofu and Bok Choy with Gingery Black Beans

■ *2500 Recipes: Everyday to Extraordinary,* by Andrew Schloss with Ken Bookman
Health Wraps
Fennel Salmon Salad Sandwich
Gorgonzola Grinders
Barley Chicken Salad
Avgolemono
Pizza Dough

Tomato, Fennel and Olive Pizza
Roasted Eggplant and Feta Pizza
Stir-Fried Brussels Sprouts
Simple Rice Pilaf
Tabbouleh with Lentils
Quinoa Pilaf

■ *Complete Book of Indian Cooking: 350 Recipes from the Regions of India,* by Suneeta Vaswani
Grilled Fish Skewers
Fish and Spinach Tenga
Crushed Potatoes with Black Sesame Seeds / Kalay Tilawalle Aloo
Garlicky Okra
Winter Greens with Split Yellow Peas / Saag aur Channa Dal
Cayenne-Spiked Apricot and Nuts Pulao

■ *300 Best Casserole Recipes,* by Tiffany Collins
Garden Vegetable Frittata
Spinach-Mushroom Quiche
Southwestern Shepherd's Pie
Chicken Florentine with Wild Rice

■ *200 Best Sheet Pan Meals: Quick and Easy Oven Recipes One Pan, No Fuss!* by Camilla V. Saulsbury
Peach Crumbles with Greek Yogurt
Three-Cheese Potato Frittata
Toasted Almond Muesli with Coconut and Chocolate
Warm Kale, Tomato, and Chickpea Salad
Crispy Baked Falafel
Roasted Salmon and Root Vegetables with Horseradish
Roast Chicken Quarters with Lemon-Dill Spring Vegetables
Broiled Halibut and Pepper Skewers with Pesto Butter Toasts
Chili-Glazed Salmon with Brussels Sprouts
Pork Tenderloin with Charred Corn Salad

■ *The Complete Leafy Greens Cookbook: 67 Leafy Greens and 250 Recipes,* by Susan Sampson
Bok Choy, Tofu and Shiitake Stir-Fry
Green Pad See Ew
Sautéed Red Chard with Lemon and Pine Nuts
Sea Salt and Chile Shanghai Bok Choy
Brussels Sprouts with Almond Thyme Butter
Garlic Herb Vinaigrette
Lemon Cumin Dressing

- *The Best Rotisserie Chicken Cookbook: Over 100 Tasty Recipes Using a Store-Bought Bird,* by Toby Amidor
Chicken and Vegetable Stew
Honey Roasted Carrots
Sheet Pan Broccoli and Cauliflower
Sautéed Zucchini with Lemon and Pine Nuts
Garlic Sautéed Spinach
Israeli Couscous and Mushrooms
Brown Rice with Peas and Carrots

- *Diabetes Create Your Plate Meal Prep Cookbook: 100 Delicious Plate-Method Recipes,* by Toby Amidor
Crunchy Peach Parfaits
Shakshuka with Chickpeas and Spinach
Pineapple-Coconut Overnight Oats
Fruit and Nut Breakfast Cookies
Whole Wheat Pasta with Spring Vegetables and Edamame
Chile Tofu and Green Beans
Roasted Sweet Potatoes
Eggplant with Tomatoes and Cumin
Red Potatoes with Chives

- *400 Best Sandwich Recipes: From Classics and Burgers to Wraps and Condiments,* by Alison Lewis
Classic Tuna Sandwich
Grilled Fish Sandwich
Chicken Waldorf Sandwich
Egg Salad with Smoked Paprika
Homemade Mayonnaise
Asian-Style Turkey Burgers
Lamb Burgers with Cucumber-Mango Raita
Veggie and Goat Cheese Wraps
Warm Italian Wraps
Chicken and Asparagus Wraps
Turkey Spinach Cobb Wraps
Classic Aïoli

- *The Best 3-Ingredient Cookbook: 100 Fast and Easy Recipes for Everyone,* by Toby Amidor
Lox Scramble
Ricotta Toast

- *200 Easy Mexican Recipes: Authentic Recipes from Burritos to Enchiladas,* by Kelley Cleary Coffeen
Chicken Mole
Red Enchilada Sauce

■ *Simply Mediterranean Cooking,* by Byron Ayanoglu and Algis Kemezys
Fettuccine with Fennel and Artichokes
Penne with Eggplants and Mushrooms
Mushroom-Spinach Lasagna with Goat Cheese

■ *The Family Immunity Cookbook: 101 Easy Recipes to Boost Health,* by Toby Amidor
Grape Oatmeal Cups
Nut and Seed Breakfast Cookies
Whole Wheat Cranberry-Orange Loaf
Lentil-Stuffed Eggplant

■ *All The Best Recipes: 300 Delicious and Extraordinary Recipes,* by Jane Rodmell
Big Batch Bran Muffins
Cheddar 'n' Chive Scones
Pumpkin Loaf
Three-Pea and Mint Salad
Southwest Slaw
Tuscan White Bean and Tomato Salad
Chickpea and Roasted Pepper Salad
Grilled Corn and Lima Bean Salad
Black-Eye Pea Salad with Tomato and Feta
Red Wine Vinaigrette

■ *Vegan Meal Prep: A 5-Week Plan with 125 Ready-to-Go Recipes,* by Robin Asbell
Quinoa Bowl with Kale and Edamame
Sesame-Miso Garlic Dressing
Tofu Sandwiches with Tomatoes, Lettuce and Avocado
Baked Marinated Tofu

■ *Up Your Veggies: Flexitarian Recipes for the Whole Family,* by Toby Amidor
Cherry, Almond and Kale Smoothie
Roasted Carrot Soup with Pesto
Crunchy Fennel Salad
All Greens Salad with Lemon Vinaigrette

■ *The Edgy Veg Easy Eats: Quick * Tasty * Vegan,* by Candice Hutchings
Higher Morels Creamy Mushroom Soup

Resources

Dr. Diana Girnita

YouTube Channel: @rheumatologistoncall

Website: https://rheumatologistoncall.com/

Blog: https://rheumatologistoncall.com/blog/

Instagram: @rheumatologistoncall

Facebook: / rheumatologistoncall

LinkedIn: / diana-girnita-md-phd-07b57810

Websites

American College of Rheumatology
https://rheumatology.org/patients/gout

National Arthritis Foundation
https://www.arthritis.org/diseases/gout

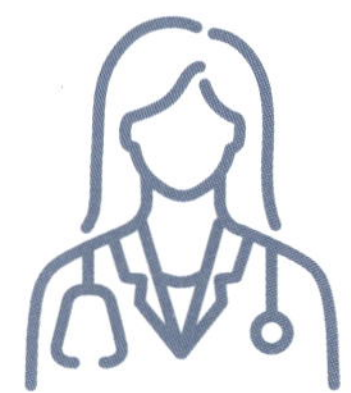

References

Chapter 1

Choi HK, Atkinson K, Karlson EW, Curhan G. Obesity, weight change, hypertension, diuretic use, and risk of gout in men: the health professionals follow-up study. *Arch Intern Med.* 2005;165(7):742–748. doi: 10.1001/archinte.165.7.742

Mattiuzzi C, Lippi G. Recent updates on worldwide gout epidemiology. *Clin Rheumatol.* 2020;39(4):1061–1063. doi: 10.1007/s10067-019-04868-9

Patron J, Serra-Cayuela A, Han B, Li C, Wishart DS. Assessing the performance of genome-wide association studies for predicting disease risk. *PLoS ONE.* 2019;14(12):e0220215. doi.org/10.1371/journal.pone.0220215

Roubenoff R, Klag MJ, Mead LA, Liang KY, Seidler AJ, Hochberg MC. Incidence and risk factors for gout in white men. *JAMA.* 1991;266(21):3004–7. https://pubmed.ncbi.nlm.nih.gov/1820473/

Zhang T, Xu X, Chang Q, Lv Y, Zhao Y, Niu K, et al. Ultraprocessed food consumption, genetic predisposition, and the risk of gout: the UK Biobank study. *Rheumatology.* 2024;63(1):165–173. doi: 10.1093/rheumatology/kead196

Chapter 2

He, Y., Xue, X., Terkeltaub, R. et. al. Association of acidic urine pH with impaired renal function in primary gout patients: a Chinese population-based cross-sectional study. *Arthritis Res Ther.* 2022;24(32). https://doi.org/10.1186/s13075-022-02725-w

Jatuworapruk K, Grainger R, Dalbeth N, Taylor WJ. Development of a prediction model for inpatient gout flares in people with comorbid gout. *Ann Rheum Dis.* 2020;79(3):418–423. doi: 10.1136/annrheumdis-2019-216277

Keenan RT. The biology of urate. *Semin Arthritis Rheum.* 2020;50(3S):S2–S10. doi: 10.1016/j.semarthrit.2020.04.007

Zhang J, Sun W, Gao F, Lu J, Li K, Xu Y, et.al. Changes of serum uric acid level during acute gout flare and related factors. *Front Endocrinol* (Lausanne). 2023;14:1077059. doi: 10.3389/fendo.2023.1077059

Chapter 3

Abhishek A, Doherty M. Education and non-pharmacological approaches for gout. *Rheumatology* (Oxford). 2018;57(suppl_1):i51–i58. doi: 10.1093/rheumatology/kex421

Bardin T, Richette P. The role of febuxostat in gout. *Curr Opin Rheumatol.* 2019;31(2):152–158. doi: 10.1097/BOR.0000000000000573

Blau LW. Cherry diet control for gout and arthritis. *Tex Rep Biol Med.* 1950;8:309–311. PMID: 14776685

Bottero V, Potashkin JA. A comparison of gene expression changes in the blood of individuals consuming diets supplemented with olives, nuts or long-chain omega-3 fatty acids. *Nutrients.* 2020 12(12):3765. doi: 10.3390/nu12123765

Brzezińska O, Styrzyński F, Makowska J, Walczak K. Role of vitamin C in prophylaxis and treatment of gout: a literature review. *Nutrients.* 2021;13(2):701. doi: 10.3390/nu13020701

Chiu THT, Liu CH, Chang CC, Lin MN, Lin CL. Vegetarian diet and risk of gout in two separate prospective cohort studies. *Clin Nutr.* 2020;39(3):837 –844. doi: 10.1016/j.clnu.2019.03.016

Choi HK, Atkinson K, Karlson EW, Willett W, Curhan G. Alcohol intake and risk of incident gout in men: a prospective study. *Lancet.* 2004;363(9417):1277–1281. doi: 10.1016/S0140-6736(04)16000-5

Choi HK, Atkinson K, Karlson EW, Willett W, Curhan G. Purine-rich foods, dairy and protein intake, and the risk of gout in men. *N Engl J Med.* 2004;350(11):1093–1103. doi: 10.1056/NEJMoa035700

Choi HK, Curhan G. Coffee, tea, and caffeine consumption and serum uric acid level: the third national health and nutrition examination survey. *Arthritis Rheum.* 2007;57(5):816–821. doi: 10.1002/art.22762

Choi HK, Liu S, Curhan G. Intake of purine-rich foods, protein, and dairy products and relationship to serum levels of uric acid: the Third National Health and Nutrition Examination Survey. *Arthritis Rheum.* 2005;52(1):283–289. doi: 10.1002/art.20761

Choi HK, Willett W, Curhan G. Coffee consumption and risk of incident gout in men: a prospective study. *Arthritis Rheum.* 2007;56(6):2049–2055. doi: 10.1002/art.22712

Clean Label Project. *Protein Powder: Our Point of View.* 2020. https://cleanlabelproject.org/protein-powder-white-paper/

Danve A, Sehra ST, Neogi T. Role of diet in hyperuricemia and gout. *Best Pract Res Clin Rheumatol.* 2021;35(4):101723. doi: 10.1016/j.berh.2021.101723

Estruch R, Ros E, Salas-Salvad J, Covas MI, Corella D, Ar s F, et al. PREDIMED study investigators: primary prevention of cardiovascular disease with a Mediterranean diet supplemented with extra-virgin olive oil or nuts. *N Engl J Med.* 2018;378(25):e34. doi: 10.1056/NEJMoa1800389

Feng Y, Duan Y, Xu Z, Lyu N, Liu F, Liang S, Zhu B. An examination of data from the American Gut Project reveals that the dominance of the genus Bifidobacterium is associated with the diversity and robustness of the gut microbiota. *Microbiologyopen.* 2019;8(12):e939. doi: 10.1002/mbo3.939

FitzGerald JD, Dalbeth N, Mikuls T, Brignardello-Petersen R, Guyatt G, Abeles AM, et al. 2020 American College of Rheumatology Guideline for the Management of Gout. *Arthritis Care Res* (Hoboken). 2020;72(6):744–760. doi:10.1002/acr.24180

Gardner CD, Trepanowski JF, Del Gobbo LC, Hauser ME, Rigdon J, Ioannidis JPA, et al. Effect of low-fat vs low-carbohydrate diet on 12-month weight loss in overweight adults and the association with genotype pattern or insulin secretion: the DIETFITS randomized clinical trial. *JAMA.* 2018;319(7):667–679. doi: 10.1001/jama.2018.0245

Georgiou K, Belev NA, Koutouratsas T, Katifelis H, Gazouli M. Gut microbiome: linking together obesity, bariatric surgery and associated clinical outcomes under a single focus. *World J Gastrointest Pathophysiol.* 2022;13(3):59–72. doi: 10.4291/wjgp.v13.i3.59

Georgoulis M, Mikhailidis DP, Panagiotakos DB. Are serum uric acid levels predictors of cardiovascular risk? An update. *Curr Opin Cardiol.* 2023;38(4):337–343. doi: 10.1097/HCO.0000000000001029

Han L, Li R, Lu J, Ren W, Ning C, Pang J, et al. Association of the Quantity, Duration, and Type of Alcohol Consumption on the Development of Gouty Tophi. *Arthritis Care Res* (Hoboken). 2023;75(5):1079–1087. doi: 10.1002/acr.24968

Hauser ME, Hartle JC, Landry MJ, Fielding-Singh P, Shih CW, Qin F, Rigdon J, Gardner CD. Association of dietary adherence and dietary quality with weight loss success among those following low-carbohydrate and low-fat diets: a secondary analysis of the DIETFITS randomized clinical trial. *Am J Clin Nutr.* 2024;119(1):174–184. doi: 10.1016/j.ajcnut.2023.10.028

Jablonski K, Young NA, Henry C, Caution K, Kalyanasundaram A, Okafor I, et al. Physical activity prevents acute inflammation in a gout model by downregulation of TLR2 on circulating neutrophils as well as inhibition of serum CXCL1 and is associated with decreased pain and inflammation in gout patients. *PLoS One.* 2020;15(10):e0237520. doi: 10.1371/journal.pone.0237520

Jacob RA, Spinozzi GM, Simon VA, Kelley DS, Prior RL, Hess-Pierce B, Kader AA. Consumption of cherries lowers plasma urate in healthy women. *J Nutr.* 2003;133:1826–1829. doi: 10.1093/jn/133.6.1826

Jakše B, Jakše B, Pajek M, Pajek J. Uric acid and plant-based nutrition. *Nutrients.* 2019;11(8):1736. doi: 10.3390/nu11081736

Juraschek SP, Gelber AC, Choi HK, Appel LJ, Miller ER 3rd. Effects of the Dietary Approaches to Stop Hypertension (DASH) Diet and sodium intake on serum uric acid. *Arthritis Rheumatol.* 2016;68(12):3002–3009. doi: 10.1002/art.39813

Juraschek SP, Simpson LM, Davis BR, Shmerling RH, Beach JL, Ishak A, Mukamal KJ. The effects of antihypertensive class on gout in older adults: secondary analysis of the Antihypertensive and Lipid-Lowering Treatment to Prevent Heart Attack Trial. *J Hypertens.* 2020;38(5):954–960. doi: 10.1097/HJH.0000000000002359

Juraschek SP, Yokose C, McCormick N, Miller ER 3rd, Appel LJ, Choi HK. Effects of dietary patterns on serum urate: results from a randomized trial of the effects of diet on hypertension. *Arthritis Rheumatol.* 2021;73(6):1014–1020. doi: 10.1002/art.41614

Kakutani-Hatayama M, Kadoya M, Okazaki H, Kurajoh M, Shoji T, Koyama H, et al. Nonpharmacological management of gout and hyperuricemia: hints for better lifestyle. *Am J Lifestyle Med.* 2015;11(4):321–329. doi: 10.1177/1559827615601973

Kontogianni MD, Chrysohoou C, Panagiotakos DB, Tsetsekou E, Zeimbekis A, Pitsavos C, Stefanadis C. Adherence to the Mediterranean diet and serum uric acid: the ATTICA study. *Scand J Rheumatol.* 2012;41(6):442–449. doi: 10.3109/03009742.2012.679964

Kontogianni MD, Chrysohoou C, Panagiotakos DB, Tsetsekou E, Zeimbekis A, Pitsavos C, Stefanadis C. Adherence to the Mediterranean diet and serum uric acid: the ATTICA study. *Scand J Rheumatol.* 2012;41(6):442–449. doi: 10.3109/03009742.2012.679964

Lu C, Li Y, Li L, Kong Y, Shi T, Xiao H, et al. Alterations of serum uric acid level and gut microbiota after Roux-en-Y gastric bypass and sleeve gastrectomy in a hyperuricemic rat model. *Obes Surg.* 2020;30(5):1799–1807. doi: 10.1007/s11695-019-04328-y

Lubawy M, Formanowicz D. High-fructose diet-induced hyperuricemia accompanying metabolic syndrome-mechanisms and dietary therapy proposals. *Int J Environ Res Public Health.* 2023;20(4):3596. doi: 10.3390/ijerph20043596

Maglio C, Peltonen M, Neovius M, Jacobson P, Jacobsson L, Rudin A, Carlsson LM. Effects of bariatric surgery on gout incidence in the Swedish Obese Subjects study: a non-randomised, prospective, controlled intervention trial. *Ann Rheum Dis.* 2017;76(4):688–693. doi: 10.1136/annrheumdis-2016-209958

Major TJ, Topless RK, Dalbeth N, Merriman TR. Evaluation of the diet wide contribution to serum urate levels: meta-analysis of population based cohorts. *BMJ*. 2018;363:k3951. doi: 10.1136/bmj.k3951

Nakagawa T, Lanaspa MA, Johnson RJ. The effects of fruit consumption in patients with hyperuricaemia or gout. *Rheumatology* (Oxford). 2019;58(7):1133–1141. doi: 10.1093/rheumatology/kez128

Neogi T, Chen C, Chaisson C, Hunter DJ, Zhang Y. *Drinking water can reduce the risk of recurrent gout attacks.* Paper presented at ACR Annual Scientific Meeting; October 16–21, 2009; Philadelphia, PA.

Nielsen SM, Bartels EM, Henriksen M, W hrens EE, Gudbergsen H, Bliddal H, Astrup A, Knop FK, Carmona L, Taylor WJ, Singh JA, Perez-Ruiz F, Kristensen LE, Christensen R. Weight loss for overweight and obese individuals with gout: a systematic review of longitudinal studies. *Ann Rheum Dis*. 2017;76(11):1870–1882. doi: 10.1136/annrheumdis-2017-211472

O'Dell JR, Brophy MT, Pillinger MH, Neogi T, Palevsky PM, Wu H, et al. Comparative effectiveness of allopurinol and febuxostat in gout management. *NEJM Evid*. 2022;1(3):10.1056/evidoa2100028. doi: 10.1056/evidoa2100028

Pitsavos C, Panagiotakos DB, Tzima N, Chrysohoou C, Economou M, Zampelas A, Stefanadis C. Adherence to the Mediterranean diet is associated with total antioxidant capacity in healthy adults: the ATTICA study. *Am J Clin Nutr*. 2005;82(3):694–699. doi: 10.1093/ajcn.82.3.694

Rai SK, Fung TT, Lu N, Keller SF, Curhan GC, Choi HK. The Dietary Approaches to Stop Hypertension (DASH) diet, Western diet, and risk of gout in men: prospective cohort study. *BMJ*. 2017;357:j1794. doi: 10.1136/bmj.j1794

Rimm EB, Appel LJ, Chiuve SE, Djouss L, Engler MB, Kris-Etherton PM, et al. Seafood Long-Chain n-3 Polyunsaturated Fatty Acids and Cardiovascular Disease: A Science Advisory from the American Heart Association. Table A1. Seafood Long-Chain Polyunsaturated Fatty Acid Composition of Commonly Consumed Seafood Varieties. *Circulation*. https://www.ahajournals.org/doi/full/10.1161/CIR.0000000000000574

Romero-Talam s H, Daigle CR, Aminian A, Corcelles R, Brethauer SA, Schauer PR. The effect of bariatric surgery on gout: a comparative study. *Surg Obes Relat Dis*. 2014;10(6):1161–1165. doi: 10.1016/j.soard.2014.02.025

Roumeliotis S, Roumeliotis A, Dounousi E, Eleftheriadis T, Liakopoulos V. Dietary antioxidant dupplements and uric acid in chronic kidney disease: a review. *Nutrients*. 2019;11(8):1911. doi: 10.3390/nu11081911

Schiavo L, Favr G, Pilone V, Rossetti G, De Sena G, Iannelli A, Barbarisi A. Low-purine diet is more effective than normal-purine diet in reducing the risk of gouty attacks after sleeve gastrectomy in patients suffering of gout before surgery: a retrospective study. *Obes Surg*. 2018;28(5):1263–1270. doi: 10.1007/s11695-017-2984-z

Singh JA, Green C, Morgan S, Sarah MD, Willig AL, Darnell B, et al. A randomized Internet-based pilot feasibility and planning study of cherry extract and diet modification in gout. *J Clin Rheumatol*. 2020;26(4):147–156. doi: 10.1097/RHU.0000000000001004

Syed AAS, Fahira A, Yang Q, Chen J, Li Z, Chen H, Shi Y. The relationship between alcohol consumption and gout: a Mendelian randomization study. *Genes* (Basel). 2022;13(4):557. doi: 10.3390/genes13040557

Teng GG, Pan A, Yuan JM, Koh WP. Food sources of protein and risk of incident gout in the Singapore Chinese Health Study. *Arthritis Rheumatol*. 2015;67(7):1933–1942. doi: 10.1002/art.39115

Tong S, Zhang P, Cheng Q, Chen M, Chen X, Wang Z et al. The role of gut microbiota in gout: Is gut microbiota a potential target for gout treatment. *Front Cell Infect Microbiol.* 2022;12:1051682. doi: 10.3389/fcimb.2022.1051682

Wang X, Qi Y, Zheng H. Dietary polyphenol, gut microbiota, and health benefits. *Antioxidants* (Basel). 2022;11(6):1212. doi: 10.3390/antiox11061212

Yamada N, Iwamoto C, Kano H, Yamaoka N, Fukuuchi T, Kaneko K, Asami Y. Evaluation of purine utilization by Lactobacillus gasseri strains with potential to decrease the absorption of food-derived purines in the human intestine. *Nucleosides Nucleotides Nucleic Acids.* 2016;35(10–12):670–676. doi: 10.1080/15257770.2015.1125000

Yokose C, McCormick N, Choi HK. Dietary and lifestyle-centered approach in gout care and prevention. *Curr Rheumatol Rep.* 2021;23(7):51. doi: 10.1007/s11926-021-01020-y

Zeng L, Deng Y, He Q, Yang K, Li J, Xiang W, et al. Safety and efficacy of probiotic supplementation in 8 types of inflammatory arthritis: a systematic review and meta-analysis of 34 randomized controlled trials. *Front Immunol.* 2022;13:961325. doi: 10.3389/fimmu.2022.961325

Zhang M, Zhang Y, Terkeltaub R, Chen C, Neogi T. Effect of dietary and supplemental omega-3 polyunsaturated fatty acids on risk of recurrent gout flares. *Arthritis Rheumatol.* 2019;71(9):1580–1586. doi: 10.1002/art.40896

Zhang Y, Chen S, Yuan M, Xu Y, Xu H. Gout and diet: a comprehensive review of mechanisms and management. *Nutrients.* 2022;14(17):3525. doi: 10.3390/nu14173525

Zhang Y, Neogi T, Chen C, Chaisson C, Hunter DJ, Choi HK. Cherry consumption and decreased risk of recurrent gout attacks. *Arthritis Rheum.* 2012;64:4004–4011. doi: 10.1002/art.34677

Zhao H, Lu Z, Lu Y. The potential of probiotics in the amelioration of hyperuricemia. *Food Funct.* 2022;13(5):2394–2414. doi: 10.1039/d1fo03206b

Chapter 4

Ingels JS, Misra R, Stewart J, Lucke-Wold B, Shawley-Brzoska S. The effect of ddherence to dietary tracking on weight loss: using HLM to model weight loss over time. *J Diabetes Res.* 2017;2017:6951495. doi: 10.1155/2017/6951495\

Index

A

ACE inhibitors, 34
Aïoli, Classic, 211
alcohol, 64, 65–67
allopurinol, 30, 53
almonds. *See also* nut butters
  Brussels Sprouts with Almond
    Thyme Butter, 217
  Cayenne-Spiked Apricot and
    Nuts Pulao, 235
  Nut and Seed Breakfast
    Cookies, 130
  Pineapple-Coconut Overnight
    Oats, 112
  Toasted Almond Muesli with
    Coconut and Chocolate, 107
  Veggie and Goat Cheese
    Wraps, 156
antioxidants, 70–71, 75
apples and apple juice
  Apple Yogurt Chia Power
    Breakfast, 113
  Baked Marinated Tofu, 153
  Chicken Waldorf Sandwich,
    137
  Crunchy Fennel Salad, 200
  Nut and Seed Breakfast
    Cookies, 130
apricots (dried)
  Cayenne-Spiked Apricot and
    Nuts Pulao, 235
  Fruit and Nut Breakfast
    Cookies, 129
arthritis, 15–17. *See also specific
    types*
arthrocentesis (synovial fluid
    analysis), 36, 38
Artichokes, Fettuccine with
    Fennel and, 186
Asian-Style Turkey Burgers, 142
asparagus
  All Greens Salad with Lemon
    Vinaigrette, 198
  Chicken and Asparagus Wraps,
    138
  Garden Vegetable Frittata,
    118
  Oven-Roasted Mixed Veggies,
    227
  Roasted Lemon Asparagus, 214
aspirin, 34
Avgolemono, 192
avocado
  All Greens Salad with Lemon
    Vinaigrette, 198
  Cornmeal Crêpes with

Avocado Filling, 124
  Pork Tenderloin with Charred
    Corn Salad, 170
  Quinoa Bowls with Kale and
    Edamame, 146
  Tofu Sandwiches with
    Tomatoes, Lettuce and
    Avocado, 152
  Turkey Spinach Cobb Wraps,
    139

B

bacon
  Turkey Spinach Cobb Wraps,
    139
bananas
  Forbidden Black Rice with
    Coconut, 110
  Fruit and Nut Breakfast
    Cookies, 129
  Peanut Butter and Banana
    Oatmeal, 111
bariatric surgery, 59–60
barley
  Barley Chicken Salad, 136
  Great Grains, Fruit and Nut
    Granola with Honey and
    Almond Butter, 106
beans. *See also* beans, green
  Cornmeal Crêpes with
    Avocado Filling (variation),
    124
  Grilled Corn and Lima Bean
    Salad, 205
  Legume and Veggie Burgers,
    178
  Quinoa Bowls with Kale and
    Edamame, 146
  Southwestern Shepherd's Pie,
    169
  Tofu and Bok Choy with
    Gingery Black Beans, 179
  Tuscan White Bean and
    Tomato Salad, 203
  Whole Wheat Pasta with
    Spring Vegetables and
    Edamame, 184
beans, green
  Chile Tofu and Green Beans,
    180
  Oven-Roasted Mixed Veggies,
    227
beef
  Southwestern Shepherd's Pie,
    169
beer, 64. *See also* alcohol

beets
  Roasted Salmon and Root
    Vegetables with Horseradish
    Sauce, 174
beverages, 64–67, 86, 116. *See
    also* alcohol
Big Batch Bran Muffins, 132
Black-Eyed Pea Salad with
    Tomato and Feta, 206
blood tests, 38
bok choy
  Bok Choy, Tofu and Shiitake
    Stir-Fry, 182
  Sea Salt and Chile Shanghai
    Bok Choy, 215
  Tofu and Bok Choy with
    Gingery Black Beans, 179
Bran Muffins, Big Batch, 132
bread (as ingredient). *See also*
    burgers; sandwiches
  Broiled Halibut and Pepper
    Skewers with Pesto Butter
    Toasts, 173
  Mushroom Bread Cups, 123
  Ricotta Toast, 125
  Shakshuka with Chickpeas and
    Spinach, 120
broccoli
  Green Pad See Ew, 183
  Pasta with Chicken and
    Vegetable Sauce, 165
  Sheet Pan Broccoli and
    Cauliflower, 216
Brussels sprouts
  Brussels Sprouts with Almond
    Thyme Butter, 217
  Chili-Glazed Salmon with
    Brussels Sprouts, 175
  Stir-Fried Brussels Sprouts, 218
bulgur
  Health Wraps, 154
  Tabbouleh with Lentils, 238
burgers, 140, 142, 178
Buttery Garlic Mashed Potatoes,
    230

C

cabbage. *See also* bok choy
  Southwest Slaw, 197
cancer, 33
cardiovascular disease, 33
carrots. *See also* vegetables
  Brown Rice with Peas and
    Carrots, 234
  Chickpea and Roasted Pepper
    Salad, 204

Ginger and Orange Braised
Carrots, 225
Health Wraps, 154
Honey Roasted Carrots, 226
Lentil-Stuffed Eggplant, 176
Roasted Carrot Soup with
Pesto, 193
Southwest Slaw, 197
cashews
Crunchy Peach Parfaits, 114
Cauliflower, Sheet Pan Broccoli
and, 216
Cayenne-Spiked Apricot and
Nuts Pulao, 235
celery. *See also* vegetables
Barley Chicken Salad, 136
Chicken Turnovers, 126
Chicken Waldorf Sandwich,
137
Classic Tuna Sandwich, 143
cheese. *See also specific types of
cheese (below)*
Chicken and Wild Rice Soup,
194
Crunchy Fennel Salad, 200
Fettuccine with Fennel and
Artichokes, 186
Gorgonzola Grinders, 155
Legume and Veggie Burgers,
178
Pork Tenderloin with Charred
Corn Salad, 170
Ricotta Toast, 125
Spinach-Mushroom Quiche,
122
Three-Cheese Potato Frittata,
119
Tomato, Fennel and Olive
Pizza, 151
Warm Italian Wraps, 158
cheese, Cheddar
Cheddar 'n' Chive Scones, 127
Chicken Florentine with Wild
Rice, 164
Southwestern Shepherd's Pie,
169
Turkey Spinach Cobb Wraps,
139
cheese, feta
Black-Eyed Pea Salad with
Tomato and Feta, 206
Grilled Corn and Lima Bean
Salad, 205
Roasted Eggplant and Feta
Pizza, 150
cheese, goat
Mushroom Bread Cups, 123
Mushroom-Spinach Lasagna
with Goat Cheese, 188
Veggie and Goat Cheese
Wraps, 156

cheese, Parmesan
Chicken and Asparagus Wraps,
138
Garden Vegetable Frittata, 118
Lentil-Stuffed Eggplant, 176
Pasta with Chicken and
Vegetable Sauce, 165
Whole Wheat Pasta with
Spring Vegetables and
Edamame, 184
chemotherapy, 34
cherries, 76–77
Cherry, Almond and Kale
Smoothie, 116
Chicken Waldorf Sandwich,
137
Crunchy Peach Parfaits, 114
Fruit and Nut Breakfast
Cookies, 129
cherry extract, 77, 78
chia seeds
Apple Yogurt Chia Power
Breakfast, 113
chicken. *See also* turkey
Barley Chicken Salad, 136
Brined and Tender Lemon
Roast Chicken, 163
Chicken and Asparagus Wraps,
138
Chicken and Vegetable Stew,
168
Chicken and Wild Rice Soup,
194
Chicken Florentine with Wild
Rice, 164
Chicken Mole, 166
Chicken Turnovers, 126
Chicken Waldorf Sandwich,
137
Pasta with Chicken and
Vegetable Sauce, 165
Roast Chicken Quarters
with Lemon-Dill Spring
Vegetables, 162
chickpeas and hummus
Chickpea and Roasted Pepper
Salad, 204
Crispy Baked Falafel, 157
Shakshuka with Chickpeas and
Spinach, 120
Veggie and Goat Cheese
Wraps, 156
Warm Kale, Tomato and
Chickpea Salad, 159
Chile Tofu and Green Beans, 180
Chili-Glazed Salmon with
Brussels Sprouts, 175
chocolate
Chicken Mole, 166
Toasted Almond Muesli with
Coconut and Chocolate, 107

chronic tophaceous gout, 40–41
cilantro
Crispy Baked Falafel, 157
Crushed Potatoes with Black
Sesame Seeds / Kalay Tilwalle
Aloo, 231
Pork Tenderloin with Charred
Corn Salad, 170
Southwestern Shepherd's Pie,
169
Southwest Slaw, 197
Citrus Fennel Slaw, 201
Classic Aïoli, 211
coconut. *See also* coconut milk
Crunchy Peach Parfaits, 114
Pineapple-Coconut Overnight
Oats, 112
Toasted Almond Muesli with
Coconut and Chocolate, 107
coconut milk
Forbidden Black Rice with
Coconut, 110
Ginger Pumpkin Soup, 195
coffee, 64
colchicine, 51
corn
Grilled Corn and Lima Bean
Salad, 205
Pork Tenderloin with Charred
Corn Salad, 170
Southwestern Shepherd's Pie,
169
Cornmeal Crêpes with Avocado
Filling, 124
couscous
Israeli Couscous and
Mushrooms, 233
CPPD (pseudogout), 16, 24
cranberries (dried)
Chicken Waldorf Sandwich,
137
Whole Wheat Cranberry-
Orange Loaf, 131
crystal-induced arthritis, 16–17,
24
CT scans, 38
cucumber
All Greens Salad with Lemon
Vinaigrette, 198
Cucumber-Mango Raita, 141
Tabbouleh with Lentils, 238
Veggie and Goat Cheese
Wraps, 156
curcumin, 87–88. *See also*
turmeric

D

dactylitis, 24, 40–41
dairy products, 81. *See also* milk
and cream; yogurt

DASH diet, 71
dates
    Cherry, Almond and Kale
        Smoothie, 116
    Date Orange Muffins, 128
dehydration, 33, 42–43, 46, 86
diabetes, 58
diet, 19, 20, 68–71
    journaling, 92–95
    meal planning, 97–98, 101
    types, 69–71, 75, 84
diuretics, 34

E

edamame
    Quinoa Bowls with Kale and
        Edamame, 146
    Whole Wheat Pasta with
        Spring Vegetables and
        Edamame, 184
eggplant
    Eggplant with Tomatoes and
        Cumin, 220
    Lentil-Stuffed Eggplant, 176
    Penne with Eggplant and
        Mushrooms, 187
    Roasted Eggplant and Feta
        Pizza, 150
    Warm Italian Wraps, 158
eggs
    Avgolemono, 192
    Classic Aïoli, 211
    Egg Salad with Smoked
        Paprika, 148
    Garden Vegetable Frittata,
        118
    Homemade Mayonnaise, 210
    Lox Scramble, 121
    Shakshuka with Chickpeas and
        Spinach, 120
    Spanish Potato Frittata, 117
    Spinach-Mushroom Quiche,
        122
    Three-Cheese Potato Frittata,
        119
    Turkey Spinach Cobb Wraps,
        139

F

fats, 82–84
febuxostat, 53
fennel (bulb)
    Citrus Fennel Slaw, 201
    Crunchy Fennel Salad, 200
    Fennel Salmon Salad
        Sandwiches, 145
    Fettuccine with Fennel and
        Artichokes, 186
    Tomato, Fennel and Olive
        Pizza, 151

fiber, 72–73
fish, 71, 83–84
    Broiled Halibut and Pepper
        Skewers with Pesto Butter
        Toasts, 173
    Chili-Glazed Salmon with
        Brussels Sprouts, 175
    Fennel Salmon Salad
        Sandwiches, 145
    Fish and Spinach Tenga, 172
    Grilled Fish Sandwich, 171
    Grilled Fish Skewers, 144
    Lox Scramble, 121
    Roasted Salmon and Root
        Vegetables with Horseradish
        Sauce, 174
flare-ups, 14–15, 25
    triggers, 45–46, 61–67
flavonoids, 73
food pyramid, 84–85
foods. See also diet; specific foods
    combinations to avoid, 67
    gout-fighting, 75–84
    protein sources, 62, 64,
        81–82
    as triggers, 61–67
    ultraprocessed, 61, 64
Forbidden Black Rice with
    Coconut, 110
fructose, 63. See also HFCS
fruit, 63, 75, 78. See also fruit,
    dried; specific fruits
    Cucumber-Mango Raita, 141
    Grape Oatmeal Cups, 108
    Pineapple-Coconut Overnight
        Oats, 112
fruit, dried
    Big Batch Bran Muffins
        (variation), 132
    Cayenne-Spiked Apricot and
        Nuts Pulao, 235
    Cherry, Almond and Kale
        Smoothie, 116
    Chicken Waldorf Sandwich,
        137
    Crunchy Peach Parfaits, 114
    Date Orange Muffins, 128
    Fruit and Nut Breakfast
        Cookies, 129
    Great Grains, Fruit and Nut
        Granola with Honey and
        Almond Butter, 106
    Nut and Seed Breakfast
        Cookies, 130
    Pumpkin Loaf, 133
    Whole Wheat Cranberry-
        Orange Loaf, 131
fruit juices, 64

G

Garden Vegetable Frittata, 118

garlic
    Buttery Garlic Mashed
        Potatoes, 230
    Classic Aïoli, 211
    Garlic Herb Vinaigrette, 208
    Garlicky Okra, 221
    Garlic Sautéed Spinach, 222
    Red Enchilada Sauce, 167
    Sesame-Miso Garlic Dressing,
        147
genetics, 19, 20, 30, 32–33
gingerroot
    Asian-Style Turkey Burgers, 142
    Bok Choy, Tofu and Shiitake
        Stir-Fry, 182
    Ginger and Orange Braised
        Carrots, 225
    Ginger Pumpkin Soup, 195
    Sesame-Miso Garlic Dressing,
        147
    Stir-Fried Brussels Sprouts, 218
    Tofu and Bok Choy with
        Gingery Black Beans, 179
    Winter Greens with Split
        Yellow Peas / Saag aur
        Channa Dal, 223
glucose, 63
Gorgonzola Grinders, 155
gout
    age and, 17–18, 19
    alcohol and, 65–67
    associated conditions, 57–61
    complications, 27, 40
    copycats of, 17, 24–25
    diagnosis of, 22–47
    diet and, 19, 20, 68–71
    flare-ups, 14–15, 25, 45–46,
        61–67
    genetics and, 19, 20, 32–33
    in history, 13–14
    lifestyle and, 18, 19, 55, 61
    managing, 21, 50–52, 90–91
    medications as cause, 33–36,
        58
    medications as treatment, 21,
        51–54
    nutrition and, 9–10, 55–56
    obesity and, 17, 18, 33, 46,
        58–61
    preventing, 49–50
    resources for, 244
    risk factors, 17–18, 19, 20,
        49–50
    self-diagnosis of, 27–28
    short-term treatments, 50–51
    tests for, 29–30, 36–38
grains, 79–80. See also specific
    grains
Grape Oatmeal Cups, 108
Great Grains, Fruit and Nut
    Granola with Honey and
    Almond Butter, 106

Green Pad See Ew, 183
greens. *See also* kale; lettuce;
    spinach
    Citrus Fennel Slaw, 201
    Egg Salad with Smoked
        Paprika, 148
    Grilled Corn and Lima Bean
        Salad, 205
    Sautéed Red Chard with
        Lemon and Pine Nuts, 219
    Southwest Slaw, 197
    Veggie and Goat Cheese
        Wraps, 156
    Winter Greens with Split
        Yellow Peas / Saag aur
        Channa Dal, 223

H

Health Wraps, 154
herbs (fresh). *See also* cilantro;
    pesto
    All Greens Salad with Lemon
        Vinaigrette, 198
    Brussels Sprouts with Almond
        Thyme Butter, 217
    Cucumber-Mango Raita, 141
    Garlic Herb Vinaigrette, 208
    Gorgonzola Grinders, 155
    Red Potatoes with Chives, 232
    Roast Chicken Quarters
        with Lemon-Dill Spring
        Vegetables, 162
    Tabbouleh with Lentils, 238
    Three-Pea and Mint Salad,
        202
HFCS (high-fructose corn
    syrup), 62–63, 64, 67
Higher Morels Creamy
    Mushroom Soup, 196
Homemade Mayonnaise, 210
honey
    Big Batch Bran Muffins, 132
    Honey Roasted Carrots, 226
    Peach Crumbles with Greek
        Yogurt, 115
Horseradish Sauce, Roasted
    Salmon and Root Vegetables
    with, 174
hot sauce (as ingredient)
    Chicken Mole, 166
    Chile Tofu and Green Beans,
        180
    Ginger Pumpkin Soup, 195
    Quinoa Bowls with Kale and
        Edamame, 146
    Tofu Sandwiches with
        Tomatoes, Lettuce and
        Avocado, 152
hypertension (high blood
    pressure), 33, 35, 58
hyperuricemia, 32–34, 74

I

imaging tests, 37–38
immunosuppressants, 35, 36
inflammation markers, 29
Israeli Couscous and
    Mushrooms, 233

J

journaling (food), 92–95

K

Kalay Tilwalle Aloo / Crushed
    Potatoes with Black Sesame
    Seeds, 231
kale
    Cherry, Almond and Kale
        Smoothie, 116
    Quinoa Bowls with Kale and
        Edamame, 146
    Warm Kale, Tomato and
        Chickpea Salad, 159
kidneys, 20, 30, 31, 33, 42–45

L

Lamb Burgers with Cucumber-
    Mango Raita, 140
Legume and Veggie Burgers, 178
lemon
    Avgolemono, 192
    Brined and Tender Lemon
        Roast Chicken, 163
    Citrus Fennel Slaw, 201
    Classic Aïoli, 211
    Lemon Cumin Dressing, 209
    Lemon Vinaigrette, 199
    Roast Chicken Quarters
        with Lemon-Dill Spring
        Vegetables, 162
    Roasted Lemon Asparagus, 214
    Sautéed Zucchini with Lemon
        and Pine Nuts, 224
lentils
    Lentil-Stuffed Eggplant, 176
    Tabbouleh with Lentils, 238
lettuce
    All Greens Salad with Lemon
        Vinaigrette, 198
    Chicken Waldorf Sandwich,
        137
    Fennel Salmon Salad
        Sandwiches, 145
    Lamb Burgers with Cucumber-
        Mango Raita, 140
    Tofu Sandwiches with
        Tomatoes, Lettuce and
        Avocado, 152
    Tuna Sandwich, Classic, 143
Lox Scramble, 121

M

mango
    Cucumber-Mango Raita, 141
maple syrup
    Grape Oatmeal Cups, 108
    Maple Cinnamon Breakfast
        Quinoa, 109
    Nut and Seed Breakfast
        Cookies, 130
    Pineapple-Coconut Overnight
        Oats, 112
    Whole Wheat Cranberry-
        Orange Loaf, 131
Mayonnaise, Homemade, 210
mayonnaise and aïoli (as
    ingredient)
    Barley Chicken Salad, 136
    Chicken and Asparagus Wraps,
        138
    Chicken Turnovers, 126
    Chicken Waldorf Sandwich,
        137
    Egg Salad with Smoked
        Paprika, 148
    Fennel Salmon Salad
        Sandwiches, 145
    Oven-Baked Sweet Potato Fries
        with Curry Mayo, 228
    Southwest Slaw, 197
    Tuna Sandwich, Classic, 143
meal plans, 97–101
meats, 62, 67, 81. *See also* chicken
    Lamb Burgers with Cucumber-
        Mango Raita, 140
    Pork Tenderloin with Charred
        Corn Salad, 170
    Southwestern Shepherd's Pie,
        169
    Turkey Spinach Cobb Wraps,
        139
medications, 21, 51–54
    and uric acid levels, 33–36,
        52–54, 58
Mediterranean diet, 69–71, 84
metabolic syndrome, 17, 26, 58
microbiome, 72–74
milk and cream, 81
    Buttery Garlic Mashed
        Potatoes, 230
    Cherry, Almond and Kale
        Smoothie, 116
    Chicken and Wild Rice Soup,
        194
    Peanut Butter and Banana
        Oatmeal, 111
    Pineapple-Coconut Overnight
        Oats, 112
    Spinach-Mushroom Quiche, 122
miso
    Sesame-Miso Garlic Dressing,
        147

mushrooms
    Bok Choy, Tofu and Shiitake
        Stir-Fry, 182
    Garden Vegetable Frittata,
        118
    Higher Morels Creamy
        Mushroom Soup, 196
    Israeli Couscous and
        Mushrooms, 233
    Legume and Veggie Burgers,
        178
    Mushroom Bread Cups, 123
    Mushroom-Spinach Lasagna
        with Goat Cheese, 188
    Penne with Eggplant and
        Mushrooms, 187
    Spinach-Mushroom Quiche,
        122

N

nephropathy, 44, 45. *See also*
    kidneys
noodles. *See* pasta and noodles
NSAIDs, 51
nut butters
    Cherry, Almond and Kale
        Smoothie, 116
    Great Grains, Fruit and Nut
        Granola with Honey and
        Almond Butter, 106
    Nut and Seed Breakfast
        Cookies, 130
    Peanut Butter and Banana
        Oatmeal, 111
nutrition, 9–10, 55–56. *See also*
    diet
nuts, 82. *See also* nut butters;
    specific nuts
    Cayenne-Spiked Apricot and
        Nuts Pulao, 235
    Crunchy Peach Parfaits, 114
    Fruit and Nut Breakfast
        Cookies, 129
    Great Grains, Fruit and Nut
        Granola with Honey and
        Almond Butter, 106
    Nut and Seed Breakfast
        Cookies, 130

O

oats
    Apple Yogurt Chia Power
        Breakfast, 113
    Crunchy Peach Parfaits, 114
    Fruit and Nut Breakfast
        Cookies, 129
    Grape Oatmeal Cups, 108
    Great Grains, Fruit and Nut
        Granola with Honey and
        Almond Butter, 106

Legume and Veggie Burgers,
    178
Nut and Seed Breakfast
    Cookies, 130
Peach Crumbles with Greek
    Yogurt, 115
Peanut Butter and Banana
    Oatmeal, 111
Pineapple-Coconut Overnight
    Oats, 112
Toasted Almond Muesli with
    Coconut and Chocolate, 107
obesity, 17, 18, 33, 46, 58–61. *See
    also* weight loss
Okra, Garlicky, 221
olive oil, 80
olives
    Black-Eyed Pea Salad with
        Tomato and Feta, 206
    Grilled Corn and Lima Bean
        Salad, 205
    Tomato, Fennel and Olive
        Pizza, 151
omega fatty acids, 82–84, 88–89
onions. *See also* vegetables
    Cayenne-Spiked Apricot and
        Nuts Pulao, 235
    Crispy Baked Falafel, 157
    Garlicky Okra, 221
    Quinoa Bowls with Kale and
        Edamame, 146
    Shakshuka with Chickpeas and
        Spinach, 120
    Warm Italian Wraps, 158
oranges and orange juice
    Citrus Fennel Slaw, 201
    Date Orange Muffins, 128
    Ginger and Orange Braised
        Carrots, 225
    Ginger Pumpkin Soup, 195
    Whole Wheat Cranberry-
        Orange Loaf, 131
osteoarthritis, 15
osteomyelitis, 25

P

parsnips
    Roasted Salmon and Root
        Vegetables with Horseradish
        Sauce, 174
pasta and noodles
    Avgolemono (variation), 192
    Fettuccine with Fennel and
        Artichokes, 186
    Green Pad See Ew, 183
    Israeli Couscous and
        Mushrooms, 233
    Mushroom-Spinach Lasagna
        with Goat Cheese, 188
    Pasta with Chicken and
        Vegetable Sauce, 165

Penne with Eggplant and
    Mushrooms, 187
Whole Wheat Pasta with
    Spring Vegetables and
    Edamame, 184
peaches
    Crunchy Peach Parfaits, 114
    Peach Crumbles with Greek
        Yogurt, 115
Peanut Butter and Banana
    Oatmeal, 111
peas, dried. *See also* chickpeas
    and hummus
    Black-Eyed Pea Salad with
        Tomato and Feta, 206
    Winter Greens with Split
        Yellow Peas / Saag aur
        Channa Dal, 223
peas, green
    All Greens Salad with Lemon
        Vinaigrette, 198
    Brown Rice with Peas and
        Carrots, 234
    Chicken and Vegetable Stew,
        168
    Three-Pea and Mint Salad,
        202
pecans
    Brussels Sprouts with Almond
        Thyme Butter (variation), 217
    Chicken Waldorf Sandwich,
        137
    Peach Crumbles with Greek
        Yogurt, 115
pegloticase, 54
peppers, bell. *See also* peppers,
    chile; vegetables
    All Greens Salad with Lemon
        Vinaigrette, 198
    Broiled Halibut and Pepper
        Skewers with Pesto Butter
        Toasts, 173
    Chickpea and Roasted Pepper
        Salad, 204
    Chile Tofu and Green Beans,
        180
    Quinoa Bowls with Kale and
        Edamame, 146
    Shakshuka with Chickpeas and
        Spinach, 120
    Tuna Sandwich, Classic
        (variation), 143
    Warm Italian Wraps, 158
peppers, chile
    Garlicky Okra, 221
    Red Enchilada Sauce, 167
    Sea Salt and Chile Shanghai
        Bok Choy, 215
    Southwest Slaw, 197
    Winter Greens with Split
        Yellow Peas / Saag aur
        Channa Dal, 223

pesto (as ingredient)
  Broiled Halibut and Pepper Skewers with Pesto Butter Toasts, 173
  Pasta with Chicken and Vegetable Sauce, 165
  Roasted Carrot Soup with Pesto, 193
Pineapple-Coconut Overnight Oats, 112
pine nuts
  Citrus Fennel Slaw, 201
  Sautéed Red Chard with Lemon and Pine Nuts, 219
  Sautéed Zucchini with Lemon and Pine Nuts, 224
pizzas, 149–51
podagra (inflamed big toe), 14
polyarticular gout, 41
polyphenols, 73, 79
Pork Tenderloin with Charred Corn Salad, 170
potatoes. *See also* vegetables
  Buttery Garlic Mashed Potatoes, 230
  Crushed Potatoes with Black Sesame Seeds / Kalay Tilwalle Aloo, 231
  Red Potatoes with Chives, 232
  Southwestern Shepherd's Pie, 169
  Spanish Potato Frittata, 117
  Three-Cheese Potato Frittata, 119
prednisone, 52
probiotics, 76
pseudogout (CPPD), 16, 24
psoriasis, 20, 33, 58
psoriatic arthritis, 16, 22, 24, 30
puff pastry
  Chicken Turnovers, 126
pumpkin
  Ginger Pumpkin Soup, 195
  Pumpkin Loaf, 133
purines, 31–32, 83

Q

quinoa
  Maple Cinnamon Breakfast Quinoa, 109
  Quinoa Bowls with Kale and Edamame, 146
  Quinoa Pilaf, 237

R

radishes
  Crunchy Fennel Salad, 200
  Roast Chicken Quarters with Lemon-Dill Spring Vegetables, 162

raisins
  Nut and Seed Breakfast Cookies, 130
  Pumpkin Loaf, 133
Red Enchilada Sauce, 167
Red Wine Vinaigrette, 207
rheumatoid arthritis, 16, 25
rice
  Avgolemono, 192
  Brown Rice with Peas and Carrots, 234
  Cayenne-Spiked Apricot and Nuts Pulao, 235
  Chicken and Wild Rice Soup, 194
  Chicken Florentine with Wild Rice, 164
  Forbidden Black Rice with Coconut, 110
  Simple Rice Pilaf, 236
Ricotta Toast, 125

S

Saag aur Channa Dal / Winter Greens with Split Yellow Peas, 223
salad dressings and sauces, 141, 147, 167, 207–11
salads, 197–206
salmon
  Chili-Glazed Salmon with Brussels Sprouts, 175
  Fennel Salmon Salad Sandwiches, 145
  Lox Scramble, 121
  Roasted Salmon and Root Vegetables with Horseradish Sauce, 174
sandwiches, 137, 143, 145, 148, 152, 155, 171
seafood, 62, 67, 71, 83–84. *See also* fish
Sea Salt and Chile Shanghai Bok Choy, 215
seeds, 82. *See also* pine nuts; tahini
  Apple Yogurt Chia Power Breakfast, 113
  Crunchy Peach Parfaits, 114
  Crushed Potatoes with Black Sesame Seeds / Kalay Tilwalle Aloo, 231
  Grape Oatmeal Cups, 108
  Great Grains, Fruit and Nut Granola with Honey and Almond Butter, 106
  Nut and Seed Breakfast Cookies, 130
  Pumpkin Loaf, 133
  Veggie and Goat Cheese Wraps, 156

septic arthritis, 24–25
sesame oil
  Baked Marinated Tofu, 153
  Bok Choy, Tofu and Shiitake Stir-Fry, 182
  Chile Tofu and Green Beans, 180
  Sesame-Miso Garlic Dressing, 147
  Tofu and Bok Choy with Gingery Black Beans, 179
Shakshuka with Chickpeas and Spinach, 120
Sheet Pan Broccoli and Cauliflower, 216
soups, 192–96
Southwestern Shepherd's Pie, 169
Southwest Slaw, 197
Spanish Potato Frittata, 117
spinach
  Chicken Florentine with Wild Rice, 164
  Fish and Spinach Tenga, 172
  Garlic Sautéed Spinach, 222
  Mushroom-Spinach Lasagna with Goat Cheese, 188
  Shakshuka with Chickpeas and Spinach, 120
  Spinach-Mushroom Quiche, 122
  Turkey Spinach Cobb Wraps, 139
  Winter Greens with Split Yellow Peas / Saag aur Channa Dal, 223
spirits, 65. *See also* alcohol
sprouts
  Health Wraps, 154
  Quinoa Bowls with Kale and Edamame, 146
  Veggie and Goat Cheese Wraps, 156
Standard American (Western-style) Diet, 69
steroids, 52
supplements, 87–89
sweet potatoes
  Oven-Baked Sweet Potato Fries with Curry Mayo, 228
  Roasted Sweet Potatoes, 229
synovial fluid analysis (arthrocentesis), 36, 38

T

Tabbouleh with Lentils, 238
tahini
  Health Wraps, 154
  Sesame-Miso Garlic Dressing, 147
  Warm Kale, Tomato and Chickpea Salad, 159

Three-Cheese Potato Frittata, 119
Three-Pea and Mint Salad, 202
tofu, 81
    Baked Marinated Tofu, 153
    Bok Choy, Tofu and Shiitake
        Stir-Fry, 182
    Chile Tofu and Green Beans,
        180
    Green Pad See Ew, 183
    Tofu and Bok Choy with
        Gingery Black Beans, 179
    Tofu Sandwiches with
        Tomatoes, Lettuce and
        Avocado, 152
tomatoes. *See also* vegetables
    Black-Eyed Pea Salad with
        Tomato and Feta, 206
    Cornmeal Crêpes with 
        Avocado Filling, 124
    Eggplant with Tomatoes and
        Cumin, 220
    Fettuccine with Fennel and
        Artichokes, 186
    Grilled Corn and Lima Bean
        Salad, 205
    Lentil-Stuffed Eggplant, 176
    Mushroom-Spinach Lasagna
        with Goat Cheese, 188
    Pasta with Chicken and
        Vegetable Sauce, 165
    Shakshuka with Chickpeas and
        Spinach, 120
    Southwestern Shepherd's Pie,
        169
    Tabbouleh with Lentils, 238
    Tofu Sandwiches with
        Tomatoes, Lettuce and
        Avocado, 152
    Tomato, Fennel and Olive
        Pizza, 151
    Tuna Sandwich, Classic, 143
    Turkey Spinach Cobb Wraps,
        139
    Tuscan White Bean and
        Tomato Salad, 203
    Warm Italian Wraps, 158
    Warm Kale, Tomato and
        Chickpea Salad, 159
tophi (uric acid crystal clusters),
    37, 38, 39–41
tortillas
    Chicken and Asparagus Wraps,
        138
    Health Wraps, 154
    Turkey Spinach Cobb Wraps,
        139
    Veggie and Goat Cheese
        Wraps, 156
    Warm Italian Wraps, 158
Tuna Sandwich, Classic, 143
turkey. *See also* chicken
    Asian-Style Turkey Burgers, 142

Turkey Spinach Cobb Wraps,
    139
turmeric, 87–88
    Crushed Potatoes with Black
        Sesame Seeds / Kalay Tilwalle
        Aloo, 231
    Fish and Spinach Tenga, 
        172
    Winter Greens with Split
        Yellow Peas / Saag aur 
        Channa Dal, 223
    Tuscan White Bean and Tomato
        Salad, 203

U

ultrasound, 37
uric acid, 31–36, 72. *See also*
    tophi
    elimination of, 31, 33
    managing, 52–54
    medications and, 21, 33–36,
        51–54, 58
    testing for, 28, 29, 30

V

vegetables (mixed), 79. *See also*
    greens; *specific vegetables*
    Chicken and Vegetable Stew,
        168
    Chicken and Wild Rice Soup,
        194
    Garden Vegetable Frittata,
        118
    Legume and Veggie Burgers,
        178
    Oven-Roasted Mixed Veggies,
        227
    Quinoa Pilaf, 237
    Roast Chicken Quarters
        with Lemon-Dill Spring
        Vegetables, 162
    Roasted Salmon and Root
        Vegetables with Horseradish
        Sauce, 174
    Veggie and Goat Cheese
        Wraps, 156
    Whole Wheat Pasta with
        Spring Vegetables and
        Edamame, 184
vitamin C, 87

W

walnuts
    Apple Yogurt Chia Power
        Breakfast, 113
    Barley Chicken Salad, 136
    Crunchy Fennel Salad, 200
    Fruit and Nut Breakfast
        Cookies, 129

    Nut and Seed Breakfast
        Cookies, 130
    Simple Rice Pilaf (variation),
        236
    Whole Wheat Pasta with
        Spring Vegetables and
        Edamame, 184
Warm Italian Wraps, 158
Warm Kale, Tomato and
    Chickpea Salad, 159
weight loss, 58–61, 70
wheat and wheat germ
    Great Grains, Fruit and Nut
        Granola with Honey and
        Almond Butter, 106
    Health Wraps, 154
    Tabbouleh with Lentils, 238
    Whole Wheat Cranberry-Orange
        Loaf, 131
    Whole Wheat Pasta with Spring
        Vegetables and Edamame,
        184
wine, 65, 67. *See also* alcohol
Winter Greens with Split Yellow
    Peas / Saag aur Channa Dal,
    223

X

x-rays, 37

Y

yogurt, 81
    Apple Yogurt Chia Power
        Breakfast, 113
    Cherry, Almond and Kale
        Smoothie, 116
    Chicken Waldorf Sandwich,
        137
    Cornmeal Crêpes with
        Avocado Filling, 124
    Cucumber-Mango Raita, 141
    Ginger Pumpkin Soup, 195
    Grilled Fish Skewers, 144
    Peach Crumbles with Greek
        Yogurt, 115
    Warm Kale, Tomato and
        Chickpea Salad, 159

Z

zucchini
    Garden Vegetable Frittata, 118
    Lentil-Stuffed Eggplant, 176
    Oven-Roasted Mixed Veggies,
        227
    Sautéed Zucchini with Lemon
        and Pine Nuts, 224
    Whole Wheat Pasta with
        Spring Vegetables and
        Edamame, 184